049614

Other Jossey-Bass books by
Seymour B. Sarason

The Creation of Settings
and the Future Societies

The Psychological Sense of Community:
Prospects for a Community Psychology

Human Services and Resource Networks:
Rationale, Possibilities, and Public Policy
(with Charles F. Carroll, Kenneth Maton,
Saul Cohen, and Elizabeth Lorentz)

The Challenge of the Resource Exchange Network:
From Concept to Action
(with Elizabeth Lorentz)

Caring
and Compassion
in Clinical Practice

Issues in the Selection,
Training, and Behavior
of Helping Professionals

Seymour B. Sarason

Foreword by Stanley F. Schneider

Caring
and Compassion
in Clinical
Practice

Jossey-Bass Publishers

San Francisco   •   London   •   1985

CARING AND COMPASSION IN CLINICAL PRACTICE:
Issues in the Selection, Training, and Behavior of Helping Professionals
by Seymour B. Sarason

Copyright © 1985 by: Jossey-Bass Inc., Publishers
433 California Street
San Francisco, California 94104
&
Jossey-Bass Limited
28 Banner Street
London EC1Y 8QE

Library of Congress Cataloging-in-Publication Data

Sarason, Seymour Bernard (date)
    Caring and compassion in clinical practice.

    (A Joint publication in the Jossey-Bass social and
behavioral science series and the Jossey-Bass health series)
    Bibliography: p. 205
    Includes index.
    1. Helping behavior. 2. Medical personnel and patient.
3. Teacher-student relationships. I. Title. II. Series:
Jossey-Bass social and behavioral science series.
III. Series: Jossey-Bass health series. [DNLM:
1. Health Manpower—standards. 2. Professional—Patient
Relations. 3. Quality of Health Care. W 21.5 S243c]
BF637.H4S27   1985   158'.3   85-14785
ISBN 0-87589-668-5 (alk. paper)

Manufactured in the United States of America

JACKET DESIGN BY WILLI BAUM

FIRST EDITION

Code 8542

A joint publication in
The Jossey-Bass
Social and Behavioral Science Series
and
The Jossey-Bass Health Series

Foreword

I was out of town when Seymour Sarason initially called me to ask if I would write a foreword to his new book. On that day, I had given an address in which I voiced great concern with many aspects of graduate education and professionalization in psychology. Repeatedly in the talk I found myself asking, "What kind of profession do we want to be?" As someone who has been closely identified with the support of graduate education and clinical training in psychology for the past twenty-two years in my position at the National Institute of Mental Health, these are not concerns I voice lightly, since they call into question major aspects of my life's work. But the need to re-examine premises comes with the job. I had quoted Sarason in my address and immediately agreed to his request when we spoke, scarcely able to conceal feelings of being delighted and honored to be asked. I eagerly awaited the manuscript.

Despite countless gems along the way, it was not until page 195 of the manuscript that the kind of question that is the essence of Sarason leapt off the paper: "What are we not thinking about that we should be thinking about but that we would not know how to think about or act in regard to, or, if we did, that would mean that we would be traveling a very lonely road?" The

The opinions expressed in this foreword are those of the author and do not necessarily reflect the opinions, official policy, or position of the National Institute of Mental Health.

uninitiated may have to read this three times, the initiated only twice. But once it sinks in, changing imperceptibly the movement of the fault lines of the mind, it is impossible not to think differently than before. This is Sarason's unique quality: to ask questions that have not been asked before, or if they have, to ask them in a new way; to bring into our awareness unattended dimensions of reality; to encourage us to recognize context and history and ask the question behind the question; and, most important, to do all of these in things that matter to people's lives.

Who else would write a book about caring? Caring is one of those unattended dimensions, a quiet attribute that enables progress even in the most difficult circumstances; but when it is absent, the most technically correct and advanced house of cards may crumble. Remarkable as it is to write about caring and compassion at all, it is even more remarkable to write about it now, when the national store of care is lavished on those who have made it. It is not that we do not care, but that we seem to have exhausted its supply for those most in need of it.

This book emphasizes a few general themes that are highly original. The reader is not likely to have perceived things in this way, if he or she has thought about them at all. Sarason circles these themes, lighting here and there with a variation, a nuance, a new insight, an elaboration that opens other doors, a personal reminiscence or vignette that makes a significant book also touching. He is very clear in stating that the book is not about what we should do (though ideas on that are inescapable) but rather how we might think about the issue that caring and compassion are largely absent from the clinical endeavor.

The scope of the clinical endeavor is surprisingly broad, since Sarason includes all activities in which a person with training and experience tries to help another person with a problem. The commonalities between medicine (with psychiatry highlighted), teaching, clinical psychology, and certain family-related aspects of law are carefully drawn, and in-depth examination of three of these professions demonstrates how the way they educate and socialize students minimizes the probability that they will be caring and compassionate, or that they will understand those who are different from themselves. Sarason's dissection of the impact of the Flexner report of 1910 on medical education is especially brilliant. Flexner's "exclusive, indeed obsessive, concern with scientific training" has had lasting effects on the selection of medical students and on medical curricula. Flexner assumed that a liberal arts education, self-selection of those with a "calling" to medicine, and exposure to mentors who presumably were caring, compassionate, and socially responsible would create caring and compassionate physicians. It is acknowledged by many people in and outside of medicine that this has occurred all too infrequently and that the situation is getting worse. A tradition of second-class citizenship for the practitioner, as opposed to the research scientist, reinforces the lack of attention to caring and compassion. Psychiatry had the best chance of overcoming the kind of clinical insularity that renders so much of medical practice uncaring, by emphasizing the dynamics of the clinical interaction. But after years of trying to gain the understanding of others through self-understanding and a briefer flirtation with the attempt to see the patient as a person in a social context, psychiatry has become "biological with a vengeance."

Clinical psychology developed out of a scientific discipline and one therefore expects that the Boulder conference, which influenced its educational and socialization requirements, would give high visibility to science, and it did. Sarason, who was a participant at Boulder, finds much more fascinating what it did *not* do, for here was the opportunity for a blueprint for a new profession, an opportunity largely missed. As Sarason points out, elements of the Boulder conference recommendations have great affinity to the Flexner report, and clinical psychology institutionalized fateful steps that would tie the field to psychiatry and the medical setting. The conference report was written without reference to anything happening in the current social milieu, and, perhaps most problematic, clinical psychology was established as an individual psychology, without regard for history, social, or familial context, and certainly with no recognition of ethnic, gender, class, or any other kind of diversity.

Psychology's greatest contributions to health, and even to

medicine as an institution, come from the fact that its perspective is *not* the usual perspective of medicine. But professionally it has legitimized itself first and foremost as a health profession, following in medicine's footsteps, and reimbursement policies will serve to bind the two even more closely together. Exclusionary battles, protection of turf, increasingly narrowed specialization, guild-serving interests—all of these have been characteristic. What happens to caring and compassion for clients when so much energy is devoted to self-protection is another matter.

More recently a few of the early deficiencies of clinical psychology have received some attention. There are finally some representatives of the various ethnic groups in graduate programs, and women are now in the majority as graduate students. If these groups were asked whether the actual graduate programs have really changed that much, they would not hail progress. The very modest level of improvement is testimony to the powerful old values. In many graduate programs, prospective clinical psychology students risked rejection if they indicated too strongly their interest in helping or caring about others or their interest to go into practice; the key to selection resided in research interests and goals.

Several of Sarason's points are so intriguing that I cannot forego some extended comment on them. They have to do with (1) the relationship of science to caring and compassion; (2) the presumed conflict between repair and prevention; (3) professionalism and the we-they dichotomy; (4) the role of education in socializing for the clinical endeavor.

A thread runs through the book that demonstrates the primacy of science and research as values in selection, education, and evaluation of students. Is science incompatible with a caring, compassionate orientation? Or, as Sarason asks, "Can we arrange a productive wedding between science and medicine [or any other clinical endeavor] without a destructive divorce between medicine and the caring, compassionate stance and action?" Sarason does not answer this question, and it still looms large. Many people think that science and humanism are incompatible. Kimble* (1984), addressing the issue for psychology, recently placed another spoke in the wheel of the two cultures argument when he affirmed, on the basis of some interesting data, that the two cultures indeed existed and that humanists and scientists showed strikingly different responses to several value propositions on a science-humanist dimension. The differences are summed up by Kimble as reflecting "a concern for a subject matter for its own sake versus 'man as the measure of all things' " (p. 839). Interestingly enough, these differences are not found in unselected groups of psychologists, but only among those who choose organizations where these values are dominant and where those who subscribe to them are further socialized in predictable ways.

Psychology has the leeway to wallow in the two cultures debate because we have not had to decide on anything important enough to force a serious confrontation of the values involved. Many nuclear physicists are no less scientific for having appreciated the need to consider the potential effects of their subject matter upon humanity. The same is increasingly true of biologists as they struggle with genetic manipulation, and it is true of a number of natural scientists who have become avid conservationists. A scientist working on the whooping crane cannot ignore the possible extinction of the object of study. In each of these instances, the awesome potential of alteration or destruction of those that are studied and/or those who study has forced moves in the humanistic direction without destroying the science. Sarason is hardly against science; the book is liberally sprinkled with suggestions for research that has not been carried out because these questions have not been asked until now. The relationship between science and caring can be seen even more clearly in the effects of understanding groups different from ourselves. Knowledge of such groups leads to a much more representative science as well as to much better prospects for caring and compassion.

*G. A. Kimble, "Psychology's Two Cultures." *American Psychologist*, 1984, *39*, 833-839.

In no single element of the book does Sarason make a greater contribution than in his iteration that the clinical endeavor presents many opportunities for prevention. Because of the narrow focus on the individual in so much clinical work, prevention possibilities are untapped. Of course, this is a Sarason dictum—the individual exists in a context of family, friends, and institutions in the larger society. When the family is considered, for example, preventive possibilities increase substantially. Sarason misses no opportunity to point out that clinical and preventive stances are not antithetical, and that it is only a narrow view of the clinical enterprise that precludes preventive activities. I find this a very congenial position and have spent a fair portion of the last two years convincing myself and trying to convince others that there is no necessary incompatibility between casualty and preventive orientations. There is no doubt in my mind that clinicians, by sheer virtue of their numbers (especially if one includes school teachers), have numerous opportunities to engage in prevention. But is narrowness of conception the only reason why this happens so rarely? We may be able better to answer that question by considering Sarason's invocation of the actor's relationship to the clinical endeavor.

Consideration of Stanislavski's methods for actors and how they might inform the clinical endeavor is as original as it is surprising. When the actor becomes the role and indeed does so with the full appreciation of the relationship of the role to all other roles in a play, Sarason believes we have a model for the development of caring and compassionate understanding of someone very different from ourselves, a model with meaning for clinical work. The actor *is* the person when this is well done; acting is replaced by being. Sarason's suggested parallels with the clinical interaction will cause not only raised eyebrows but an accusation of violation of the first tenet of a clinical relationship—thou shalt not muddy the boundaries between clinician and client. But how do we really get to understand another person in context, to be caring and compassionate? Can this be done with strict objectivity, and if it cannot, how can we be certain that any blurring is in the client's, rather than the clinician's, interest? And are there we-they distinctions that precede

these; are professionals educated and socialized in ways that enhance feelings of distance from, or superiority over, clients?
How many things protect professionals from becoming involved
or from needing to care? Are incentives in the system designed
to promote caring, or to maximize technological applications?
These are a few of the questions that lead me to be less than
sanguine about a great rapprochement between clinical and preventive endeavors.

Prevention, especially primary prevention, forces identity
questions on clinicians. Since the populations in primary prevention are not sick, diagnosed, or labeled, they are not patients. Do people who are not patients require doctors or clinicians? Similar questions arise in community-based participatory
prevention research, where distinctions between subjects and
experimenter tend to vanish. The professional's knowledge remains pertinent, but the personal equation is changed. What effects, if any, do such relationships in primary prevention have
on caring?

Sarason points out frequently that professional and graduate education do not prepare clinicians who are caring, compassionate people. In psychology, at least, graduate and professional education is due for an overhaul, and I suspect the
situation is no different in related fields. In fact, while many
old deficiencies remain, such as the paucity of meaningful instruction in ethnic- and gender-related material, students now
think about professional education mainly as the ticket to licensure. Rather than education informing and improving practice,
licensing and credentialling requirements fuel the educational
process. Overspecialization is another characteristic that further
narrows professional (and scientific) education.

I must forego comment on several other thoughtful points
made in this book, not the least of which shows the clinician as
much the victim as the client. The question finally emerges:
"What kind of person do we want the clinician to be and how
do we help such a person become that?" It is a question not unlike the one I reported asking myself at the beginning of this
foreword. Sarason and I would welcome similar questions from
others, since they will tell us someone is paying attention.

Sarason watchers will need no recommendation to read this book; the news that it is written will be sufficient. The book deserves the widest audience throughout the entire field of human services, among people who are supposed to care and the many who think they do. It is really a gentle, even intimate, essay. No individual is blamed, but the cumulative effect is shattering. When the manuscript arrived, two pages were missing. I have not received them, so I have something to look forward to as well, for there is not a page in this book from which one cannot learn something.

July 1985   Stanley F. Schneider
                                                            National Institute of
                                                            Mental Health
                                                            Rockville, Maryland

Preface

I have been in and around the clinical scene for more than forty
years, during an era that witnessed not only unprecedented
growth in the traditional clinical professions but the emergence
of new ones as well. I was both a participant in and an observer
of this growth, a proponent as well as an antagonist. One part of
me wanted to believe that growth meant progress; at the same
time another part inchoately sensed that we were paying a high
price for quick and dramatic growth. We know a good deal
about human behavior in different contexts, and one of the
things we know is that we are pretty poor at managing quick
growth, whether it be the growth of an organization or of a profession. The reasons are many, both practical and theoretical,
but one of the most worrisome is that coping with quick growth
short-circuits thinking, analysis, and reflection. We make a virtue of necessity, point ourselves to a foreshortened future, and
regard understanding the past as a luxury we cannot afford. The
societal pressure to grow, and to grow quickly to meet escalat-
ing needs—and that is precisely the societal pressure the clinical
professions experienced during and after World War II—implicitly conveyed the message that these professions were basically
sound except that they had to learn how to train more practitioners. This is not to say that the clinical professions did not
undergo change. Change they did, but more in regard to their
theories and less in regard to whom they selected, how the se-

lection was made, the characteristics of training sites, and the rites of passage testifying to a minimally acceptable level of competence for independent practice. So, for example, when you contrast psychiatry before World War II to psychiatry during the two decades following the war, you observe a dramatic change from a biological to a psychoanalytic orientation. That was an important change, a very influential one, but it hardly altered in any significant way the relation between psychiatry and the rest of medicine, the range of training experience, the rationale for supervision, who did the supervision, and, as I indicated earlier, who was selected (and in what ways) into the profession. The biological and psychoanalytic psychiatrists explained and treated personal disorders in very different but overlapping ways, but one of the things about which they were in full agreement was that they were psychiatrists; that is, they had very similar backgrounds and experiences in medical school and in speciality training. In the past two decades the pendulum has swung back, and the biological orientation has again become the regnant orientation.

Another factor besides quick growth helps prevent a truly radical examination of the basis of a profession's educational rationale: professionals are not noted for their willingness to engage in self-scrutiny. It is to stimulate such self-scrutiny that I have written this book. Such self-scrutiny should always be at the top of the agenda because, as this book attempts to demonstrate, when professionals are required by internal and external pressures to engage in self-scrutiny they tend to come up with recommendations that confirm the maxim that the more things change the more they remain the same. So, today, we are witnessing internal and external pressures for change in medical and allied professions in response to a perceived marked dilution in the qualities of caring and compassion among clinicians. Although those pressures are not new, they seem stronger and more widespread, especially among the general public who resent being treated as objects and not as persons. I was spurred to write this book by my feeling that not only were the issues surrounding caring and compassion becoming more poignant and urgent but the proffered remedies were at best of the

Band-Aid variety and at worst guarantors of disappointment, much as has been the case in the past when these issues have periodically surfaced. But another factor also stimulated the writing of this book: the current discussion about caring and compassion focuses exclusively on medical clinicians, totally ignoring the professionals outside the medical arena who also fulfill a clinical role. In terms of the public interest, can we afford to ignore these other clinicians? Are the issues surrounding caring and compassion less worrisome in these nonmedical professions? My experience led me to answer both questions in the negative.

The themes central to this book have been germinating in me for a number of years. Indeed, they first began to take shape (although the word *shape* conveys a degree of order that is misleading) when Esther Sarason and I were clinical psychologists in a new state institution for the mentally retarded during World War II. Esther was then, as now, a most caring and compassionate clinician, always unwilling to excuse any practice or rule that interfered with actions consistent with her understanding of the quantity and quality of help an individual required. I tended to be more "practical," a euphemism too frequently used to justify not fully discharging the obligation to be caring and compassionate.

When I came to Yale to direct its graduate program in clinical psychology, I was required to become acquainted with diverse types of clinicians populating the medical scene. In addition to graduate students in psychology, I taught medical students, nurses, and psychiatric residents. More important, I was exposed to the world view that dominated medical education and practice. There was much I found upsetting about that world view, not the least of which was how that world view rendered the clinician insensitive to the phenomenology of the ill person, the familial-social context without which the clinician's understanding of the person is egregiously incomplete. This world view focuses on the patient; all else is relegated to the background. However well intentioned that focus may be, I was forced to conclude that, not only is it so inordinately narrow that it frequently and literally causes problems for the patient's relatives, but it arbitrarily and effectively divorces the clinical from the preventive stance.

However immersed I was in the clinical scene, I managed to sustain on a continuous basis my interest in the public schools. This took a variety of forms, in all of which I came to know and work with teachers, administrators, school psychologists, counselors, and school social workers. And when in the late fifties Burton Blatt, another example of what caring and compassion means in action, came to head up the special education department at Southern Connecticut State University in New Haven, he made it possible for both of us to alter the style, substance, and goals of teacher training in that department. During those years I came to see what I should have seen long before: teachers are clinicians, and however that conflicts with the popular imagery of a teacher in a classroom, it does not conflict with the everyday fact that teachers must always fulfill the role of helper to personally or academically distressed children. The medical and educational scenes had a lot in common, but in neither were the interrelationships among understanding, caring, and compassion squarely recognized and confronted.

The more I pondered my experiences in the medical and educational arenas, the more I began to see that these interrelationships were central to many professions and that our over-learned habit of viewing professions differently because they have different labels had become, however historically understandable, an obstacle to clarity, and a constraint upon point of view and appropriate action. Physicians, psychiatrists, clinical psychologists, teachers, and lawyers—these were professionals for whom the issues surrounding caring and compassion could and had to be posed. These issues are no less present in many other clinical professions, but these are the five professions I know best; and if I devote more pages to the physician, it is because these issues have been most clearly posed with regard to the physician's practice. I devote an entire chapter to Flexner's historic 1910 report on medical education for two reasons. First, it was a dramatically catalytic force for change. Second, it glossed over all of the issues surrounding caring and compassion in those in helping roles. Indeed, it was only when I scrutinized

that report in light of subsequent public and professional concerns about physician behavior that I came to see that the problems were by no means peculiar only to physicians.

As the issues began to take shape, I found myself success-
fully resisting starting to write. For one thing, I would be writing about several professions, each of which has a unique history and, on the surface at least, very different goals and roles.
Doing justice to one is no mean task, to take them all on
seemed overwhelming. It is one thing to say that a particular
profession has experienced dramatic growth and very mixed social consequences; it is quite another to describe that growth
and relate it in concrete ways to issues of caring and compassion. Furthermore, caring and compassion are "murky" concepts having much the same status that St. Augustine gave to
time: "What is time? If no one asks me, I know what it is. If I
wish to explain to him who asks me, I do not know." In addition, the empirical literature on the nature and consequences of
caring and compassion (their presence or absence) is amazingly
sparse, however crucial the two qualities are regarded by (apparently) everyone. As someone said decades ago about psychotherapy, "Psychotherapy is an undefined technique applied to
unspecified problems with unpredictable outcome. For this
technique we recommend rigorous training."

Two developments made it possible for me to start writing. One was the realization that I had been viewing this book as
a scholarly one in which I would put the issues and the relevant
literature in a broad social, historical, institutional, educational
framework that would give appropriate attention to what we
know and highlight the areas of ignorance future investigators
should seek to illuminate. What I had at first failed to appreciate was that these issues had hardly been posed, let alone systematically studied, and that what I needed to do was to present the issues as clearly as I could so that it would not be easy
to dismiss or ignore them. This meant explaining why we must
enlarge our view of the scope of the clinical endeavor, why the
issues surrounding caring and compassion have not been realistically confronted, what the obstacles (psychological, educational, institutional) to caring and compassionate actions are,

and, most important, what the obligation to be caring and compassionate requires of us, clinician and nonclinician alike.

The other factor that propelled me to start writing was reading in the *New York Times* of September 13, 1983, about a forthcoming report by the Association of American Medical Colleges, a report offering remedies that would counter the tendency in physicians to be less caring and compassionate than they should be. When I read that report, with a sinking heart, with that "here we go again" feeling, I knew that I had to get started.

So the major aim in this book is to state and examine the possibility that caring and compassion among clinicians in various professions are qualities that are in short supply. I say "possibility" because there is little firm evidence on the nature and extent of the problem, despite the fact that many observers, now and in the past, have been critical of these professions. It is both puzzling and upsetting that these qualities—surely central to the clinical endeavor—have not been studied, even though billions of research dollars have been expended to improve the quality and outcomes of clinical service. It is an omission that can no longer be justified. My own experience forced me to conclude that the problem is of serious dimensions and can only get worse. I run the risk, as do others, of being seen as unduly pessimistic. I will be more than satisfied if the reader, after finishing this book, agrees that the issues are real and deserve far more discussion and study than they have received. And my satisfaction will be dramatically increased if the reader comes to see that the issues concern a variety of fields we ordinarily do not think of as "clinical."

Initially, this book was entitled "Caring in America: A Critique of the Clinical Endeavor." That title derived from my conviction that the clinical endeavor exists and always will exist in a transactional relationship with the larger society, reflecting and in turn affecting features of the society in which it is embedded. Another virtue of that initial title was that it suggested that the problem did not inhere in the personality of individuals but in a society having a distinctive history. I very much wanted to avoid appearing to criticize, let alone to make scapegoats of, individuals. No clinician wants to be, or intends to be, uncaring and uncompassionate. But it became apparent in the course of writing that the initial title promised far more than would be delivered. I mention this change here to stress that what I have to say should not be interpreted as referring to an individual psychology, because such an interpretation would, in my opinion, be another instance of blaming the victim. Book titles, like professional labels, both obscure and illuminate.

From these aims it follows that this book is intended for two audiences. The first is heterogeneous only on the surface: physicians in general, psychiatrists, clinical psychologists, teachers, and lawyers. They are the clinicians I discuss, and the ones I know best. They have far more in common than their labels suggest. The other audience is indeed heterogeneous: they are the recipients of clinical services and, far more than the first audience, they are aware of their need for caring and compassion and are concerned when that need is not met. Indeed, it is my impression that in the past twenty-five years hardly a month has gone by without some publication by a consumer of clinical services describing frustration and resentment at dealing with this or that clinician, and if you include novels, the number of these publications discernibly increases.

Acknowledgments

The extent of my indebtedness to Esther Sarason I have already noted, and although I would love to elaborate on the substance of that debt, I shall refrain from doing so if only to keep peace in the house. And I have much the same to say about Burton Blatt whose capacity for caring and compassionate actions is well known to countless people around the nation.

I am fortunate to have many dear friends. At a crucial time in the writing of this book, when it seemed that finishing it would be delayed, one of those friends, Elizabeth Lorentz, demonstrated by her actions what caring and compassion meant. I hope these three friends regard this book as partial repayment for what they have given to me. I wish also to express my gratitude to Yale University in general, and its Institution for Social and Policy Studies in particular, for creating the conditions that make thinking and writing not tasks you struggle with on weekends but a normal part of daily living.

New Haven, Connecticut   Seymour B. Sarason
July 1985

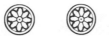

Contents

The Author

Seymour B. Sarason is professor of psychology in the department of psychology and at the Institution for Social and Policy Studies at Yale University. He founded, in 1962, and directed, until 1970, the Yale Psycho-Educational Clinic, one of the first research and training sites in community psychology. He received his Ph.D. from Clark University in 1942 and holds honorary doctorates from Syracuse University and Queens College. He has received an award for distinguished contributions to the public interest and several awards from the divisions of clinical and community psychology of the American Psychological Association, as well as two awards from the American Association on Mental Deficiency.

Sarason is the author of numerous books and articles and has made contributions in such fields as mental retardation, culture and personality, projective techniques, teacher training, the school culture, and anxiety in children.

To Esther
with my thanks and love

Caring
and Compassion
in Clinical Practice

Issues in the Selection,
Training, and Behavior
of Helping Professionals

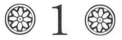

1

Introduction
to Issues and Problems

In this introductory chapter, I try to give the reader a feel for the major themes that will run through this book. This I do as much to alert the reader to the boundaries within which I discuss issues as to avoid arousing expectations that I offer concrete remedies. It is understandable if each of us in regard to a troublesome public issue impinging on our lives asks: What should we do? That, in regard to the issues discussed in this book, is in one sense premature, because we are proceeding on the basis of little or no secure knowledge. It is not premature in the sense that, faced with issues that affect all of us, we, like the professional clinician, act on the basis of what knowledge we have and what our values require us to try despite awareness of our ignorance. So although this book is not about what we should do, implications for actions will not be hard to discern.

The interpersonal qualities that characterize the discharging of a clinical service are no less important to judge than the outcome itself. No one, least of all the recipients of the service, have to be reminded of the importance of outcomes, and scores of thousands of journals and books have been devoted to the assessment of outcomes. But, comparatively speaking, the assessment of the means by which these outcomes have been achieved has been ignored. And by *means* I do not refer to technical procedures bur rather to the qualities of the interpersonal transactions between clinician and client. So, for example, within the past few years, individuals and groups within the medical community have articulated concern that medical schools are graduating increasing numbers of physicians in whom the caring and compassionate stance is absent. It is a concern shared by many in the general public, and it has long been a subject for novels, the theater, and published accounts by patients' spouses and families of their experiences with physicians and medical settings. At the same time that we are told in the various mass media about the scientific and technical advances in medicine—and they are indisputable—we are also being told that we are paying a price that should not be glossed over. But what is the price? As best as I can determine from these published accounts and reports, it is that uncaring and uncompassionate behavior violates two ideals. The first of these ideals says that physicians owe sick and troubled people a sensitive understanding and responsiveness that go beyond the presenting symptoms to include the phenomenological plight of the individual. This is not an ideal of courtesy or noblesse oblige but rather of a willing giving and using of oneself for the purposes of understanding the individual-familial-social context in which illness is always embedded, an understanding that informs caring and compassionate actions. The second of these ideals goes far beyond the medical one and, indeed, antedates it in that it speaks to what should characterize any meaningful encounter between two people. What we expect of the physician-patient relationship is a derivative of the ideal relationship between people. The Hippocratic ideal cannot be separated from that described by Plato, Socrates, and Aristotle. If the patient-physician relationship has distinctive features, that is no warrant for concluding that these features are or should be seen as unique in human relationships. It is in terms of these ideals that the perceived increase in uncaring and uncompassionate actions among physicians has become a matter of concern to some medical educators who cannot be accused of being unknowledgeable or utopians or bleeding hearts. It should be noted that their published concerns have not been criticized by anyone within or without the medical community. Their concerns have struck responsive chords.

    The two ideals do not fully explain why these concerns have surfaced and coalesced with such clarity in recent decades.

Two additional and interrelated factors are in the picture, if only as unarticulated background. The first is the perception of the adverse consequences of the seemingly inexorable growth of large organizations in all spheres of our society, a growth in which everything, public and private, seems to become related to everything else, and the individual at the foot of this mountainous growth is wondering what is going on in the Kafkaesque castle at the top. We have been made familiar with this growth in the private sector and federal and state governments, but we have been less familiar with the fact that this kind of metastatic growth has become no less a feature of the health sector in its public and private manifestations. To an unprecedented degree, the physician has become the organization man or woman familiar with the dilemmas of being an agent with divided loyalties between client and organization, a dilemma too frequently resolved by excusing uncaring and uncompassionate behavior. The second and related factor is the poignancy with which people in all segments of society strive unsuccessfully to experience that sense of intimacy, that sense of community, that sense that others respect and seek to understand you, that feeling that someone else cares. In regard to physicians, we need not try to determine whether in "the good old days" they were more caring and compassionate than the physicians are today. Myth or fact, that is what people believe to have been the case. It is not the case today, and that is a belief widely shared within and without the medical community. Increasingly, the physician is seen as insensitive, uncaring, uncompassionate, unwilling or unable to discharge the caring function. In brief, the current concern is about the dilution of the strength of millennia-old ideals in a world in which the individual, client or physician, tends to feel impotent and dissatisfied. The physician no less than the client is a victim of societal transformations that are distinguishing characteristics of the modern world. What has happened in medicine is disturbing because it indicates that the societal transformations that have become so problematic for so many people have intruded into a relationship in which caring and compassion have been, on the level of rhetoric at least, treasured, distinguished features.

But, a critic can argue, how do we "really" know that

there is a basis for these concerns about the behavior of physicians? Granted, the critic can continue, that caring and compassion should be quintessential features of the physician's makeup, should we not refrain from a blunderbuss-like indictment
until we have more secure evidence that there is a problem? The
fact is that (as we shall see later) neither I nor the authors of reports on medical education are criticizing individuals; rather, we
are criticizing a state of affairs in which physicians are socialized
and educated and from which they are catapulted into another
state of affairs that reinforces interpersonally impoverishing
stances. Furthermore, is it not strange—I would say both inexcusable and revealing—that, although these concerns are
about features of the physician-patient relationship that everyone says is crucial, they have for all practical purposes gone unstudied despite the billions of research dollars that have been
poured into the medical community in the post–World War II
era? I do not think this is happenstance, nor do I regard it as a
conspiracy of silence, but rather as a reflection of the tendency
to take for granted that verbal adherence to ideals leads to actions consistent with those ideals; that is, a confusion between
intention and outcome that would not be tolerated elsewhere in
the research endeavor. The critic is right to ask for hard data,
but in their absence, and in the presence of the fact that no one
has contradicted those who voice concern, and because these
concerns are the opposite of trivial to the public welfare, the
call for remedial action is quite understandable. There is another part to the answer: I know of no conception or theory of
modern society—its origins, vicissitudes, and dynamics—that
would not predict that the field of medicine would take on features of the larger society in which it was embedded. What
would require explanation would be if medicine had withstood
taking on the coloration of its surround. It always took on the
coloration of its surround, but now that coloration intrudes
into our awareness, because it offends us. Finally, the critic
should pay more attention to proposed actions than to the basis
or object of criticism, because the proposals for change are (unfortunately) modest and unlikely to have anything like a significant impact.

The concern about the personal styles and qualities of medical clinicians deserves attention, study, and experimentation. However, precisely because the problem has been identified in medicine, it is very likely that we will continue to be blind to the fact that it is a problem by no means peculiar to that field. The hallmark of the clinical endeavor is that one person tries to do his or her best, on the basis of training and experience, to help another person with a problem. The clinical interaction is a face-to-face encounter between a troubled individual and someone who has formal credentials to help in regard to whatever the presenting problem may be. Just as there are physicians who are not clinicians—who do not deal directly with troubled individuals—there are clinicians who are not physicians. For example, there is no classroom teacher who is not faced with troubled children and parents whom the teacher is expected to help. Ordinarily, we do not think of teachers as clinicians; the imagery conjured up by the labels *teacher* and *educator* is that of someone standing up and instructing seated students in a classroom asking them questions, evaluating their work, and stimulating and sustaining their interest. It is imagery that is grossly incomplete and misleading, as any teacher will attest. Similarly, we do not think of lawyers as clinicians, although in any one day thousands of lawyers are in the role of helping troubled individuals traversing the psychological and legal minefield of divorce, troubled as individuals and as parents. And, like teachers, they know well that the problems brought to them go far beyond the legal and have percolating consequences in the present and the future. If teachers and lawyers are not perceived as clinicians, it says less about the realities of their roles and more about our victimization by labels.

We must overcome our narrow conception of who is in the clinical endeavor, but one reason requires mention here. The clinical endeavor is time consuming, its "cure rate" far from the ideal, and its financial costs to individuals and society expensive and ever increasing. It has been said that clinicians spend most of their time as carers, not as curers, a fact that should occasion no surprise when one considers that they are dealing with problems that already exist, frequently with a degree of complexity and seriousness that sets drastic limits to efforts of repair. No one disputes the assertion that the prevention of problems is incomparably more desirable than trying to repair their consequences. What opportunities for prevention are there in an endeavor focused on problems that are manifest? The standard answer is that the clinician seeks to prevent secondary and tertiary consequences, that is, to contain the problem, to prevent things from getting worse. Far more often than not, that answer is associated with imagery of a single, troubled individual. But, as clinician and client alike know full well, the problem of the individual is always embedded in and has actual and potential effects on that person's familial-social network of relationships. The problems brought to the clinician, any type of clinician, are or can become problems for others with whom he or she is related. The problem may be cancer, a failure in school, or divorce, but it is never a problem of, in, or on a single individual. In practice, unfortunately, the problem is too frequently labeled, conceptualized, and treated as an individual problem. Imagine the situation where we can videotape a large, random sample of clinical interactions. What opportunities for prevention (primary, secondary, and tertiary) could we discern in regard to the individual and those who are or likely will be affected by the presenting problem? That question has hardly been asked and studied, a reflection of the narrow training of clinicians as well as of the tendency to see prevention and repair as polarities.

When you examine how clinicians are trained, it becomes obvious that, despite the lip service paid to prevention, the emphasis in practice is on the presenting problem conceived in the most narrow ways. As a result, myriad opportunities for prevention are not seen, or they are glossed over, or their neglect is excused by "practical" considerations such as lack of time or by variants of the statement: "I do not deal with those issues, they belong to somebody else, it is not in my clinical ball park." It is precisely because the clinical endeavor presents so many opportunities for prevention—and nothing rivals prevention for desirable consequences—that it is so important to recognize how unrealistic and impractical it is to restrict the label *clinical* to medical and allied fields. Resources are always limited, and how we allocate them reflects not only dominant values, ideologies, and power-political alignments but the influence of traditional ways of defining problems and professional roles. Nowhere are these traditional ways better exemplified than in the restricted ways we have been taught to apply the label *clinical* and to accept in practice the arbitrary separation of the clinical and preventive endeavor.

In this book, I shall be talking about physicians in general, psychiatrists in particular; clinical psychologists; teachers; and lawyers. There are other professions I could have included, but my choices were governed by the fact that, in over forty years in and around the clinical community (as a clinical and community psychologist in and out of the university), I have come to know some professions better than others. And if I spend more pages in this book on medical and allied fields, it is because issues surrounding caring and compassion have more often been raised in relation to these fields. There is also another reason for this emphasis: the explanations for the perceived dilution of the caring and compassionate stance among medical clinicians largely involve the substance, pressures, and ambience of medical school education and medical practice. But these explanations are discouragingly ahistorical. Why did medical schools become the pressure cookers they are, the "trade schools" in which the student is so absorbed with the accumulation of fact and technique that he or she sees no difference between a person and a symptom? (As a friend said after he came home from the hospital: "To my doctor I was a gall bladder, to the radiologist I was an X ray, to the lab technician I was blood, to some nurses I was a pain in the neck, to the medical student I was a bunch of facts she had to record, and to the admissions and discharge office I was Blue Cross–Blue Shield. I didn't know what a many-splendored thing I was.")

To understand how this state of affairs developed is no easy matter, and I do not attempt a comprehensive answer, but I do concentrate on a document that was crucially fateful for American medicine. I refer, of course, to Abraham Flexner's 1910 report on medical education in the United States and

Canada (Flexner [1910], 1960). Although Flexner sought to wed medicine to science, he was never in doubt that more fundamental to the clinical endeavor than scientific knowledge and research was the clinician's ability to have the kind of understanding of the plight of patient and family that made appropriate caring and compassionate actions possible. But how do we instill such understanding in the prospective physician? In one paragraph, Flexner raises the question, says it is a very difficult question, and concludes that the best guarantee that the physician will have these qualities is a liberal arts education, to become what he called "the educated man." If I spend many pages on Flexner's report, it is because his solution is identical to proposed remedies offered today. But even if one looks at the problem historically, there is the possibility that explanations in terms of that history, though they may have a surface plausibility, may still in whole or in part be wrong. If these explanations are correct, then caring and compassion should be less problematic in other fields (for example, psychology, law, education), where the deficiencies of medical education are absent. This is the kind of cross-field comparison I undertake. At the least, what emerges from this comparison is that, whatever the benefits of a liberal arts education, and they are many, producing caring and compassionate people is not among them. It is not the first time hope is confused with accomplishment, intention with action.

It will become apparent that from my perspective there is no reason to be optimistic that the concerns being voiced today will make much of a difference. For one thing, riveting only on medical fields unduly narrows our understanding, if only because it simply fails to recognize how many nonmedical fields involve the clinical endeavor. Second, the history of curriculum reform in and outside of medicine does not permit one to entertain high hopes. Third, the criteria by which people are selected to enter a clinical field (again, any clinical field) are irrelevant, perhaps counterproductive, to the goal of selecting individuals who have the potential to become caring and compassionate clinicians. It says a lot that not only are training centers in our universities loath (somewhat of an understatement) to alter and literally to experiment with selection criteria, but there is for all practical purposes no research, certainly no systematic research, on this issue in selection, despite the billions of dollars that have poured into research on the clinical endeavor. Fourth, as long as we continue to talk about caring and compassion as attitudes, we make it too easy to ignore the tenuous and complex relationship between attitude and action. When I use the words *caring* and *compassion* in later pages, I refer to caring and compassionate actions, in the spirit of the talmudic caveat: you will be judged by what you do, not by what you say is in your heart. Fifth, any meaningful remedial proposal requires changes in the behavioral and programmatic regularities of the settings in which clinicians are trained, something the curriculum reformers have almost always vastly underestimated as sources of obstacles to change—for example, confusing their passion and purpose with those of the bulk of others in the setting, which rarely if ever is warranted. Sixth, how one person helps another to act caringly and compassionately has hardly been discussed, the prepotent response being that supervision must become better and mentors have to be models of such actions to the student. As will become apparent, I do not disparage supervision, but my experience prevents me from being satisfied with the recommendations that we must increase supervisory time, as if the pressures on supervisory time were a major reason for the relative lack of focus on the issues surrounding caring and compassion.

Terms such as *caring* and *compassion* have an obvious ring of virtue to us. No one regards him- or herself as uncaring and uncompassionate, and no one wants to be regarded as such by others. And, however much we may agree on defining these terms, that agreement noticeably lessens when we are asked or required to judge whether the action of one person toward another has these features. Instructive in this regard, as later pages will indicate, is how perceptions of clinicians change when they or members of their families become patients; that is, on the receiving end of the clinical endeavor. It is an unsettling experience, because, often for the first time, they are forced to become aware of the obstacles that make caring and compassionate

behavior a sometime thing in the clinical endeavor. It is an illuminating experience. And it is precisely for the purposes of
illumination, not solution, that I discuss a nonclinical profession
for which caring and compassion is the central issue because it
requires each of its members to understand another person in
his or her complexity, to *become* that other person even if that
person is wildly different in values, style, actions, and purposes
from the one seeking understanding. It is an understanding that
is impossible unless one is prepared to be caring and compassionate. I refer to actors in the theater—more specifically, to the
conceptualization of acting by the Russian director Stanislavski.
If I discuss his conceptualization for the purpose of illuminating
the nature of caring and compassion—the predictable obstacles
that stand in the way of being caring and compassionate—it is
because I believe that what he says and proposes is relevant to
the clinical endeavor and that we cannot ignore his contribution. How we absorb it and how we try to apply it will depend
on many things beyond the scope of this book. That it illuminates aspects of the clinical endeavor in an amazingly refreshing
way, I have no doubt. At the very least, it is another instance of
how surface differences among fields obscure fascinating underlying similarities.

I entreat the reader, in reading the chapters that follow,
to control—better yet, to avoid—the reaction that I am blaming
or criticizing individuals, that I am saying that this clinician is
bad and that one is good. Aside from the fact that I do not regard the issues as reflecting the motivations and lacks of individuals—as if anyone wants to be, wittingly or unwittingly, uncompassionate—there is the danger that the reader may see the
issues in terms of the personality of individuals. That is a danger
for the reader whose experiences lead him or her either to agree
or to disagree with what I say or describe. That there are clinicians who are caring and compassionate goes without saying. Indeed, as I shall emphasize, explanations for the decrease of caring and compassion among those in the clinical endeavor avoid
the question: How does one account for clinicians who are caring and compassionate? The reader who finds himself or herself disagreeing with what I say and describe because it is dis-

crepant with his or her experience cannot ignore the fact that, both within and without the clinical endeavor, people see it otherwise and explain it in nonindividual terms. The issues surrounding caring and compassion in the clinical endeavor are not new ones. What is new is the perception that the issues have taken on a scope and urgency that demand discussion, study, and remediation. I share that perception, recognizing that hard data are lacking, a lack that in itself speaks volumes. I will be more than satisfied if this book contributes to the effort to gain wider currency for these issues than is presently the case. These are not professional issues in the usual sense. They are issues for everyone.

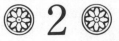

Scope of the Problem: Relation of Institutional Context and Clinician Behavior

I came to visit my mother in her hospital room a week after she had been operated on for lymphatic cancer, a major site of which was behind the thyroid gland. Speech was impossible for her, because of both the surgery and an emergency tracheotomy two days later. We had been told that there might be temporary interference with speech. When I entered her room, she was crying and visibly agitated. I called the nurse, who could offer no explanation. Finally, my mother indicated that she wanted pencil and paper. The message she wrote said that, just before I had arrived, the surgeon had appeared, accompanied by several interns and residents. He explained to his younger colleagues my mother's condition, the type of surgery that had been performed, and that it had been necessary to sever several major vocal chords—following which he and the others left the room. That was how my mother found out that she would never talk above a whisper.

A second anecdote involved me as a patient. I had to go through an hour-and-a-half procedure that continuously "filmed" the activity of my heart. It was a painless, indeed fascinating, experience. Fascination aside, I was anxious about what the procedure would indicate. That was a Wednesday morning. I was told that it would take one or two days for the computer analysis of the filmed record and results to be placed in the hands of the cardiologist. Having heard nothing by the next Tuesday morning, I phoned the cardiologist's office and was told by the nurse: "Didn't they phone to tell you that there had been a malfunction in the computer and that another procedure would be necessary?" Angry, I called the radiologist's office and was told that they had called my home but no one had answered. Why, I asked, did they not call my office, the number for which I had given them? And why did they not try to get me over the weekend? I should also add that in the several different radiological procedures that were done, I never saw the radiologist, but I assume that he or she or they existed.

Two more anecdotes. Minutes after a mother has delivered her child, and still groggy and dazed from the experience, she is told that her child has mongolism (Down's syndrome). The second instance is that of a mother who had come for the first time to a pediatric clinic a few weeks after delivery; in the hall she meets her doctor, who, in the process of saying hello and continuing down the hall, tells her that her child is mentally retarded. Both instances took place in a prestigious medical center in 1976. Having been intimately involved in the field of mental retardation for over forty years, I can assure the reader that these instances are only somewhat extreme.

The final instance, which will allow me to put the others in perspective, concerns the film version of *One Flew over the Cuckoo's Nest*. As I was viewing the film, I found myself caught between two strongly conflicting reactions. On the one hand, I was gripped by the artistry with which the struggle between McMurphy and the hospital in general, and Miss Ratched in particular, was developed. I indulged my disdain, indeed hatred, of nurse Ratched and my somewhat grudging admiration and respect for antihero McMurphy. I reacted internally with violence to the violence to which this patient was subjected. I have had enough experience with mental institutions to know that what Dorothea Dix described to the Massachusetts legislature in

1848, what Dr. Burton Blatt described to the same legislature in 1968, and what Dr. George Albee wrote in reaction to Frederic Wiseman's state hospital film, *Titicut Follies,* is well encapsulated in *One Flew over the Cuckoo's Nest.* (The reader should consult Blatt's 1970 book *Exodus from Pandemonium,* written after a stint as deputy commissioner in Massachusetts's Department of Mental Health.) And yet, as I watched the film, I got increasingly upset by what I thought would be the central message viewers would carry away with them: that this was an interpersonal drama about two very different kinds of people locked in a tragic, one-sided battle. In short, if either or both of them had been different kinds of persons, the tragedy would not have occurred. From my standpoint, that view was an example of a fact obscuring a truth. And that truth, very briefly, had several interrelated components:

1. The state hospital was organized and staffed in ways that for all practical purposes gave decision-making power on the wards to those (nurses and aides) who spend the most time with patients. Those professionals (psychiatrists and administrators) vested with ultimate powers of decision, and presumably possessing more sophisticated knowledge and skills, spend the least time with patients on the ward; they are essentially consultants who appear at certain times or are on call, and they are dependent on what ward personnel describe to them. Why the hospital is organized in this way—the historical, economic, and professional considerations from which such an administrative structure emerged—is never alluded to. Why such a structure maximizes misinformation and inappropriate treatment actions recedes as an issue as the focus remains on the personality clash between McMurphy and Ratched. That this clash is but one instance of clashes that such a structure guarantees on wards is not an issue the film takes up.

2. The state hospital is part of and under the control of a state mental health department that formulates and implements policies, allocates resources, and in diverse ways affects each hospital and agency under its jurisdiction. In short, what we see in the film is in part a reflection of people, policies, and decisions made elsewhere. The next point provides one example.

3. One scene in the film takes place in the office of the superintendent of the hospital. It is a meeting of the top administrative and professional staff, and the agenda is McMurphy: what to do with and about him. One of the participants is Asian, the others Caucasian. Let us leave aside the fact that having one "foreigner" at the meeting is a gross misrepresentation of the percentage of foreign physicians in most state hospitals. What cannot be put aside is that the participants are an unimpressive lot: smug, unquestioning, unimaginative, and concerned only with law and order. The criteria by which these participants were hired for their positions in the hospital, the salaries and perquisites they are given, the definition of their duties and responsibilities, the criteria by which they are evaluated for promotion and salary increases—in regard to all of these and more, the staff of the central office in the mental health department in the state capitol are crucial initiators, overseers, and judges. One cannot understand what one sees in the film apart from the relationship between this particular hospital and the state department of mental health. It is ironic that, just as McMurphy is portrayed as combating and subverting a stultifying, uncaring staff and ambience, that is precisely the way the administrative-professional staff in many state hospitals experience their relationships to the central office in the state capitol. And just as McMurphy is ground into submission to the powers that be, that is also the frequent fate of those whom the central office selects to care for the McMurphys of the world. But let us not scapegoat the central office, because they describe much the same feelings and experience in their relationship to the governor's office, the legislature, and an uncomprehending public. The McMurphy-Ratched struggle *is* interpersonal, it is the stuff of tragic drama, but the "lessons" one draws about preventing such struggles must take account of far more than the phenomenology of the interpersonal.

The film does not address the question—nor was it addressed by the many nonprofessionals whom I informally interviewed about their reactions to the film—of how people are selected for positions in the state hospital. (As I indicated earlier, the criteria for and jurisdiction over personnel selections are not

by any means the primary prerogative of the local hospital.)
The fact is that the concept and process of selection are hardly
appropriate in these instances. That is only somewhat more true
in the case of the nonprofessional than it is of the professional
staff. Two features have long characterized personnel selection
in these hospitals: the willingness of people to work in them
and the most superficial criteria for employment—criteria that
have never been demonstrated to be at all correlated with interpersonal sensitivity, the caring attitude, or competence to deal
patiently and nonpunitively with myriad goads to the less at-
tractive capabilities of the human organism. If Miss Ratched and
other staff members were employees of that hospital, it said
more about self-selection than it did about selection by the hospital, the central office, or the state personnel department. If
there are large numbers of foreign staff in these hospitals, it is
because these hospitals have rarely been in the position of selecting. (There is a difference between selecting and employing.)
I should also point out that the large number of foreign staff in
these hospitals is very much related to longstanding features,
policies, and attitudes of American medicine in general and psychiatry in particular.

These comments are not intended as criticisms of the
film. I am not suggesting that the film should have addressed
these points or should have been more didactic. I am also aware
that in this Greek-like tragedy in which the end is contained in
the beginning—the gods (the hospital) will have their way—more
is implied than that this is an interpersonal drama; for example,
that the hospital is a crazy place, and not all of the craziness
resides in patients. As a work of art, it is a superb film in the
way it presents us with the interpersonal struggle in a physically
encapsulated place. However, its artistic excellence should not
obscure the fact that, from my standpoint, the film has the intended consequence of reinforcing the view, only partially valid,
that the tragedy was the making of individuals and, therefore,
the solution is in substituting "good" people for "bad" people,
caring people for insensitive people. Miss Ratched, my mother's
surgeon, the two physicians who related in the way they did the
diagnosis of mental retardation to parents—when one sees or

hears about such people, the prepotent tendency is to blame the kinds of people they are. Change the actors, and the scripts will lead to less upsetting outcomes. And when, as is likely, you reflect on that tendency and concede that these people are not willing sadists luxuriating in their ability to cause misery, you probably will conclude that faulty selection and ineffective training are the factors that need to be changed. Those are understandable and reasonable conclusions, but I must stress the fact that, precisely because they emphasize the characteristics of people, they obscure the significances of the social-educational contexts from which these professionals have come, the contexts into which they have come to learn their trade, and the contexts in which they practice what they have learned. Just as the McMurphy-Ratched conflict cannot be understood apart from the institutional, professional, political, economic, administrative context—a context rooted in a history that continues to pervade the present—we cannot ignore the role of similar contexts in which changes in selection and training are recommended. You can change training educational curricula and criteria for selection, but the sought-for benefits of those changes can be achieved only if the larger context in which these changes take place does not work at cross-purposes to those changes.

There is a built-in problem here. We can literally see things and people; for example, we see McMurphy, Ratched, and others alone or in relation to each other in visually graspable places. But you cannot see what I have called contexts, what others might call systems. Concepts such as context or system are inventions of the human mind; they have a different status from words that refer to a thing (for example, a stone) or a person (McMurphy). Precisely because we can see people and identify with their actions and inferred feelings, we attribute to them causation and explanation that ignore the role of context or system. As a consequence, when these actions elicit in us a need to intervene in, ameliorate, or change an observed iniquitous state of affairs, it takes the direction of altering people's actions or substituting "good" for "bad" people. Context or system remains untouched. This has long been a characteristic of efforts to improve mental hospitals, just as it has long been a characteristic that exposés of these hospitals recur with amazing regularity in the public media and judicial system.

So, as I indicated, in 1848, Dorothea Dix presented to the Massachusetts legislature her historic address on the inhumane conditions in that state's "humane" institutions. Miss Dix had only words at her disposal, not still pictures or a film, but one can assume that her descriptions had effects similar to those experienced by the viewers of *One Flew over the Cuckoo's Nest*. Somewhat more than a century later, Dr. Burton Blatt, reminding another assembled Massachusetts legislature of Miss Dix's address, presented similar descriptions, with pictures (Blatt, 1970). And those intervening decades did not lack for exposés of similar conditions in that state's hospitals. Massachusetts, of course, was by no means atypical in this regard. Each exposé led (and leads) to public chagrin, uproar, and outrage, with the resolve to get rid of those who condoned or were themselves guilty of brutality in its diverse guises. Locate the individual culprits, bring in new, more caring people, perhaps beautify the surround somewhat, move everyone and everything into new quarters, or introduce an in-service training program, and sin will be eradicated once and for all time. The interval between exposés is sufficiently long, given short memories and the ahistorical stance in these matters, to obscure the possibility that the problem does not reside exclusively in the perverse motivations and personality peculiarities of individuals. We can see and document brutality, we can identify individuals in whom the caring attitude appears to be nonexistent, we can point to administrative-professional practices or rules that place individuals at risk, and morally we cannot ignore these factors or fail to deal with them. But, as the historical record demonstrates, when we deal with these factors as if they are only, or even largely, explainable and resolvable in terms of personality characteristics, we assuage our consciences at the expense of recognizing the characteristics of the larger context or system in which the individuals we see are a very small part of a cast of a drama taking place on a much larger stage, a stage we can never literally see but that we have to conceptualize and invent.

Still another example of the cyclical concern for the lack of caring in the clinical endeavor is an article by Nelson (1983) in the *New York Times*. The headline of the article, on the first page of the science section, is: "Can Doctors Learn Warmth?" The subheadline reads: "Concern over lack of compassion leads to nationwide action." Here are the first three paragraphs of the article:

> Leading American medical professors and physicians are moving to correct what they regard as a serious problem in their profession: a lack of compassion in the treatment of patients.
>
> "There is a groundswell in American medicine, this desire to encourage more ethical and humanistic concerns in physicians," Dr. John A. Benson, Jr., president of the American Board of Internal Medicine, said in a recent interview. "After the technological progress that medicine made in the 60's and 70's, this is a swing of the pendulum back to the fact that we are doctors, and that we can do a lot better then we are doing now."
>
> The movement is centered in medical schools, where, some experts believe students can be dehumanized, and even brutalized, by the experience. Medical students are often physically and mentally overwhelmed by the demands placed upon them. They sometimes observe inhumane treatment of patients, and they themselves are not infrequently treated as ciphers by those above them in the medical hierarchy. As a result, these young would-be doctors begin, in turn, to view troublesome patients as ciphers.

The article then lists and discusses steps taken by the Association of Medical Colleges "to reassert the importance of compassion in the practice of medicine." (The verb *reassert* is well taken, because these "view with alarm" articles appear every ten years or so, their contents having predictable similarities.) First, a series of hearings were held around the country to pinpoint "lapses in the humanity of medical education." Second, educational programs emphasizing values, ethics, and compassion have been adopted in many medical schools. Third, medical certification boards are to give increased weight "to humanistic qualities in devising examinations and in monitoring the education of specialists." Fourth, there is an ongoing three-year study on the entire content of medical education. The article correctly notes that, although "doubts about whether physicians spend enough time caring for patients have been voiced for centuries," recent developments have exacerbated these doubts—for example, growth of specialization, third-party payments, exponential increase of and dependence on new and complex technology, and the ambience and process of medical education: socialization into the profession.[1]

If I view the developments described in the article without enthusiasm or optimism, it is not because of any nihilistic or cynical proclivity on my part. There is a difference between pessimism rooted in temperament and that rooted in the actuarial basis provided by social history. Of course, one should take satisfaction, indeed pride, in the knowledge that there are people in the clinical professions who have the courage to be "whistleblowers," to say out loud that the emperor may not only be naked but may also have a serious disease. But when whistleblowing has the consequence of eliciting actions based on the wrong diagnosis—or on a conception of etiology discernibly invalid or demonstrably superficial—one may be pardoned if, with sinking heart, one finds oneself concluding: "Here we go again." Although I shall have more to say about this in later chapters, the concerns articulated in the article avoid confronting several questions. First, why have past efforts

---

[1]The report of the Association of American Medical Colleges (1984) entitled *Physicians for the Twenty-First Century*, was published several months after the *New York Times* article; the report lacks the passion of the newspaper article. The knowledgeable reader, reading on and between the lines, will readily grasp the seriousness of the concerns, but the report is not likely to convey to other readers the sense of urgency and crisis the newspaper article communicates.

to make physicians more compassionate been ineffective—indeed, why has the situation become worse? Second, to what extent do the criteria for selecting people for medical careers take account of "compassion"? Third, is it possible that these criteria work at cross-purposes to the goal of selecting people high on the characteristic of compassion? Fourth, are the contexts of socialization (medical school, internship-residency) ones in which the characteristic of compassion gets diluted or even extinguished? In short, are we dealing with a situation and proposed remedies in no way genotypically different from what I discussed earlier in regard to the film *One Flew over the Cuckoo's Nest*?

The issues are not peculiar to a state hospital or to medical education; they are issues that arise whenever and wherever major societal institutions appear to be intractable to change in ways that society deems desirable. Today, for example, we are bombarded with reports critical of public education and containing remedies that are intended to improve the atmosphere and outcomes of schooling. As in the case of the current concerns of medical educators, the authors of these reports judge schools to be so seriously flawed as to imperil the public welfare—that is, if allowed to continue, these situations will inexorably have an adverse impact on the social fabric. There is another similarity (Sarason, 1983): in both instances, there is almost total amnesia for the historical fact that the reports of today are amazingly like those of previous decades. There is one interesting and instructive dissimilarity. Whereas colleges of education have rarely, if ever, been in a situation of truly selecting people for the profession, medical schools have long had such a large pool of candidates from which to choose that they have steadily raised what they consider to be appropriate criteria for selection. And yet, despite such a large pool, these criteria have to no one's satisfaction led to more compassionate physicians. The skeptic could suggest that, if colleges of education were in a position to employ intellectual and educational criteria similar in principle and even substance to those used by medical schools (that is, very high grade average from highly respected schools, high test scores on the Graduate Record Examination, and so on), we might well end up with future reports that are carbon copies of those of today and the past. On what basis do we call someone a skeptic because he or she sees no compelling evidence that the criteria are relevant for the selection of the kinds of people the profession and the larger society say they want? If the critics of education are clear about anything—and they are clear about few things—it is that entrants to the profession have to be more carefully selected, and I would guess that they would be ecstatic at the prospect of colleges of education employing the standards of educational and intellectual performance used by medical schools. Critics of medical education have always been gun-shy about facing the possibility that their criteria for selection play an important role in producing the problem of "lack of compassion." In fact, there has been less change in the process and criteria of selection of medical students than in any other aspect of medical training.

There is one more similarity between criticisms of public and medical education, a similarity that is far more serious than the critics realize in that it raises the "intractability" question: can our purposes be realized within the context of the existing social structure and value system of our public and medical schools? Have these purposes in the past not been realized for the same reasons? If the answer to the first question is even a qualified "no," and to the second question even a qualified "yes," then the situation is indeed serious, in that we are conceding that the problem is intractable in the existing contexts. The similarity can be put this way: Granted that we may not be selecting by the most appropriate criteria and procedures. But even if we selected more appropriately, we still have to face the fact that, as soon as the person begins the socialization process into teaching and medicine, that person encounters an ambience, a set of pressures, a hierarchy of values on the basis of which one is judged worthy or unworthy, that literally change the person's outlook and actions in undesirable ways. In the case of public education, the critic is referring to what the aspiring professional experiences in his or her training and in the culture of our schools, experiences that are frequently infantilizing, stultifying, and destructive of the spark of creativity and of the dynamisms of hope and motivation. If that sounds extreme, it is because one has not listened to the critics from within and without the educational arena. The disdain with which the critics talk about the quality of the preparation of educational personnel in schools of education and about what life is like in our schools—and the amount of disdain expressed publicly is pale compared to what is said privately—is enough to give the most dedicated students cause for rethinking career goals. And it is no different in the case of the critic of medical education who, on and between the lines, is drawing a picture of the medical school and hospital as akin to a jungle in which student-eating faculty and supervisors—driven by ambition, competitiveness, and the insatiable thirst for scientific knowledge, fame, and survival—turn the compassionate student into the noncompassionate clinician, a process always, of course, articulated and cloaked in the garments of efficiency, objectivity, necessity, and a presumed superior level of morality.

What the critics of these two societal institutions seem not to recognize is that they are describing contexts of socialization inimical to their goals of change, just as they were inimical to those in the past with similar goals. And when I say *inimical,* I mean that these contexts are intractable to the sought-for change, that, whatever the degree of change that will be accomplished, it will be very small, transient, and promptly forgotten even when a decade or so later the same viewing with alarm will take place. As I said earlier, one should be grateful that there are people who bring the issues to the social agenda. But the real significance of their role today inheres in their claim that the situation is not the same as before but worse. Whether or not the situation has deteriorated and will continue to do so—the existing "evidence" would not stand up in the courts of science—should not obscure the fact that many knowledgeable people believe that to be the case. And in the case of medical education and practice, I refer not only to many medical educators but to a significant portion of the general population to whom the adjective *compassion* does not readily come to mind when they reflect over their experiences with hospitals, physicians, and the allied professions.

There is irony in the fact that the concerns of medical educators about the lack of compassion are implicitly, and sometimes explicitly, based on a conception of the "social contagion of disease." Let me illustrate this point by an example from public education, another instance of parallelism between these two social arenas. The example concerns the Head Start program, which was initiated by President Lyndon Johnson in the sixties with much fanfare. Beginning as it did in the sizzling sixties, that program, which initially was a summer program, is not explainable outside of the sensitivities stimulated by racial conflict, the civil rights movement, and the war on poverty. There was one other major factor: the overwhelming evidence that socially and economically disadvantaged children, black and white, did poorly in our schools. The preschool Head Start program was intended as a way of preventing later school failure. That was the surface rationale. What did not get stated was the widely held view that the schools to which children from these strata went were inadequate on many grounds for normal passage by them through the grades; that is, their educational difficulties inhered less in any intellectual or social deficits and more in unstimulating, noncompassionate, unsupportive school environments, where the social atmosphere and substance of the curriculum extinguished rather than reinforced curiosity and interest.

Put in another way: Head Start was to be a kind of inoculation against catching the disease of educational arrest that was so catchable or contagious in our schools. It did not take long before it became apparent that this preschool inoculation would need booster shots once the children entered school, and such shots took the form of a "follow-through" program. There is evidence (Zigler and Valentine, 1979; Sarason and Klaber, 1985) that Head Start and comparable programs may have had, on average, the desired effects, although these effects are by no means robust. No dispassionate (or, for that matter, passionate) advocate for Head Start has claimed that the school setting has altered significantly in the direction of being a very positive plus in the educational development of Head Start children. Quite relevant for my later purposes in this book is Zigler's chapter (Zigler and Valentine, 1979, p. 495) in *Project Head Start: Success or Failure?* Zigler was one of the forces behind Head Start and the first director of the Office of Child Development, into which Head Start was later placed. If anything is clear in that chapter, it is Zigler's plea that Head Start be viewed not from society's traditionally narrow criteria of adequate intellectual and educational performance but from that of the consequences of *caring actions* that dilute or prevent discomfort or misery or support social competency. Listen to Zigler's concluding statement:

> How many dollars is it worth to head off a case of measles? To raise the measured IQ by 10 points by the end of a program? To reduce a child's wariness of strange adults? To discover that the presence of Head Start in a community led to the provision of more health and educational services to all economically disadvantaged children? Or to demonstrate that a child was given a set of experiences that clearly improved the quality of his life for that one year he had them? As one of the creators of the Head Start program and the public official who was at one time responsible for its management, I readily admit that I have been more influenced by the positive than by the negative findings concerning the value of Head Start. By the same token, in the absence of specific, identifiable dollar gains, I prefer to attribute a high rather than a low figure to Head Start's identifiable accomplishments. This is to admit no more than that even sophisticated readers of evaluation studies must finally introduce some of their own values before drawing a conclusion as to whether a program is worthwhile or not.

To evaluate Head Start primarily by the values dominant in the school culture is to restrict or downgrade dramatically the range of possible caring actions. There is, unfortunately, absolutely no reason to believe that the stance on which the caring actions informing Head Start are based have been assimilated into the school culture. This is not because school personnel are heartless or uncaring people—they are not—but because the school culture and the process by which people are socialized into that culture define and justify ends and means in very narrow ways. So, when I say that the school is intractable to the stance underlying Head Start, it is less a criticism than it is calling attention to the possibility that we are asking of the school something to which it is unable to accommodate. If that conclusion is correct, even in part if not in whole, it requires us to give up the tendency to see institutional change primarily in terms of altering the motivations of individuals or of demonstration projects intended to be so persuasive as to compel observers (assuming they have observed, which is rarely the case) to undergo conversion. In my experience in public schools and medical schools, demonstration projects initiated explicitly for the purpose of conversion—to convert the "primitives," so to speak—begin and end as alien bodies, fated to leave no trace in institutional memory.

     Nowhere today in discussion of their concerns do medical educators recognize the possibility that the culture of the medical school and hospital may be lethal to change by the efforts they have chosen. And yet they describe an atmosphere and ideology so powerful and encompassing, so successful in defeating all past similar efforts, that it should occasion no surprise if the medical student and neophyte catch the disease of "lack of compassion." What would require explanation would be if the outcome were otherwise. I first became aware of this situation forty years ago, when I was a member of a small child-guidance unit in Yale's Department of Pediatrics. That unit was remarkable on two counts: it may have been the first of its kind in such a department, and it was headed by Dr. Edith Jackson, a well-known child psychoanalyst. In those days (the unit began before World War II), it was rare, and probably unique, that a psychoanalyst would have an important teaching position anywhere in a medical school. Soon after I joined the unit, I was made aware of how alien that unit was in the department. To put it succinctly, the goals of that unit were precisely those enunciated by the medical educators in the *New York Times* article of September 13, 1983 (Nelson, 1983)—almost forty years from the day I joined the unit.

Although the unit provided service primarily to children in the hospital or those referred from the outpatient clinic, its existence was justified as a teaching site for medical students, interns, and residents. To teach what? To teach understanding of and compassion for the psychological status of sick children and their families; put in another way: to enlarge the horizons of medical personnel about the dilution and prevention of misery attendant to the psychological trauma of hospitalization; to aid them to see that they had the responsibility to treat more than the physical condition; and to get them to understand that to pigeonhole the psychological and physical into distinct categories was to have the most restricted of views of "healing" and that to care for someone's well-being required sensitivity to and compassion for that being's social psychological state and context. There was no hard sell, if only because Edie Jackson was incapable of it. The hard-sell approach would have brought out into the open attitudes destructive of whatever surface courtesy and respect this unit enjoyed.

One such attitude was that whatever this unit did—and to members and students in the department, the goals of the unit had the characteristics of an inkblot—was in no way central to the field of *medicine*. And by *central* I mean that, if the unit was suddenly to disappear, there would be few if any mourners at the memorial service. Another attitude was that the techniques and practices employed in the unit did not meet the criteria of scientific validity and that there was no evidence that outcomes had scientific credibility. Finally, there was an attitude as influential as it was both subtle and disquieting to those who held it: Yes, what this unit wants us to understand and act on is very important, should be taken very seriously, and we need more of it if we are to become comfortable with it, but we have no *time* for it in either our training or our practice. To those (few) medical students and interns who had this attitude, what the unit stood for was a necessity that had the attributes of an unpurchasable luxury. To those (even fewer) residents and faculty members who shared this attitude, what the unit stood for was important only for those who wanted to specialize in matters psychological; it was necessary for them, but not for those seeking a career in "scientific medicine" and overwhelmed by the pressures such a career entailed. There was no disposition to recognize that the argument based on time constraints reflected a hierarchy of values and unreflectively justified specialization of role and function.

It was extraordinarily difficult for those of us in the unit to adjust to the fact that we were second- or third-class citizens in an institution devoted to the repair and prevention of the human misery that so often attends and surrounds illness. But, if it was difficult, it was not because of our need for status but because our conception of caring took far more into account than does the traditional conception of repair. I remember once saying to a faculty member in pediatrics that the unit of treatment should be not the child but the family.[2] He looked at me as if I had just plumbed the depths of nonsense and then, in all seriousness, with only a trace of asperity, said: "Those who are not real physicians will never understand why medicine has made as much progress as it has."

I have heard that argument over the years, an argument that contains a kernel of truth coated with a glaze of rationalization. The most extreme example of this attitude was expressed by a former undergraduate student who had gone into pediatrics, had married, and together with his wife was visiting me in my office. At one point, he said that one of the real pluses in their marriage was that they were both physicians, "and only physicians can live with and talk to physicians." He said this

---

[2] I joined the unit on a part-time basis at the same time that I held a position as psychologist at a new state training school for mentally retarded individuals. It was in that institution that I quickly learned that trying to understand and help children independent of their families made neither theoretical nor practical sense. That is a point I have emphasized, somewhat monotonously, perhaps, over the decades (for example, Sarason, 1949, 1985; Sarason and Doris, 1979), increasing acceptance of the position existing side by side with very little change in practices.

with complete and smug seriousness, unaware that he had indicted his own inability to understand and live with "foreign-
ers," which included, I shall assume, many, if not all, of his patients. It is one thing to claim distinctiveness; it is quite another
thing to confuse it with uniqueness. What is unusual in this
example is not what this young man said to me. Physicians say
that to each other all the time, as any half-candid physician
and a voluminous literature (literary and scientific) will attest.
What was unusual was that he said it to me, just as it would
have been unusual if I had said to him how bad I felt that as a
physician he would never understand—*could* never understand
—what it was like to be a psychologist! To which he could have
retorted with a smile: "But everybody is a psychologist of
sorts." Is there anyone who is not a physician of sorts?

Another related fragment of autobiography: Beginning in
the early forties, Dr. Jackson began to push for creating a rooming-in unit in obstetrics, where the newborn would be with the
mother throughout the hospital stay. At the core of the rationale
for such a unit was the belief that the physical separation of
mother from the newborn was upsetting and anxiety arousing
for the mother and, furthermore, postponed and interfered with
the processes of mutual adaptation between mother and infant
(and between father and infant). This was a rationale that reflected caring and compassion in two related ways: the way the
physician understood and responded to the mother's feelings
and concerns and the way the mother wanted to express her
caring and compassion for her newborn. It was not a rationale
considered appropriate for all mothers but only for those who
expressed such a desire. The reactions to the proposal were predictable and of three kinds. The first was that the idea was the
latest of a long line of examples of misguided sentimentality, as
well as of the unctuous mystification of the importance of the
mother-newborn relationship. The second was that, since there
was no "real" evidence that traditional practice was medically
and psychologically deleterious to mother and infant, why try
something new that might turn out to have adverse effects? The
third reaction had many components, but they all had one root:
resistance to the changes (leadership, administrative, role) that

would obviously have to take place. It would take a book of modest size to describe what happened over several years before the rooming-in unit was able to be opened (and it was a *very* small unit). There were many times in that before-the-beginning period when the advocates for the unit were ready to give up, unable to cope with the political and interpersonal warfare. It would be correct but incomplete to explain what happened only in terms of the reaction of setting, any setting, to significant change, because that would neglect the fact that the internecine warfare circled around two issues: the centrality given to caring and compassion in the original rationale and then, as discussions got under way, how caring and compassion would get reflected behaviorally in the running of the unit. If everyone was crystal clear that the quality and style of interaction between staff and parents on the unit would be different, they were far from agreement about what that would actually mean in practice.

But, one could ask, does not the fact that the unit came into existence say something positive about the tractability of the medical school hospital setting to an altered view of caring and compassion? And, from the vantage point of the passage of four decades, how does one explain accommodation of the setting to comparable rationales—for example, fathers participating in the delivery process? In regard to the rooming-in unit (as well as to the child-guidance unit), I must make mention of an individual who in his everyday relationships with everyone was quintessentially the caring and compassionate person, in terms not of what he said but of what he did. He was also the head of Yale's department of pediatrics and a towering figure nationally in that field. If that department had a child psychoanalyst on its staff, if it had a child-guidance unit, if a rooming-in unit came into existence, it said as much about Dr. Grover Powers's caring, compassionate personality and behavior as it did about his political status. For Grover Powers, no medical treatment could ignore the needs, wishes, and attitudes of the patient and family. The patient was not a body, period. If Dr. Powers could listen to Dr. Jackson, it was not only because he was a courteous and respectful person but also because what she espoused struck a responsive chord in him. And he well knew that in supporting her efforts he could count on his faculty to be tolerant but not truly supportive. If, like Dr. Jackson, he was willing to swim against the tide, it was because of inner conviction and not because either was sanguine about discernibly affecting the tide.

And that is the point: whatever the child-guidance and rooming-in units stood for in regard to patient-clinician relationships, it had predictably little of a percolating effect within the larger setting. If rooming-in and comparable programs have become more frequent in the post–World War II era, it is largely because federal monies became available for their implementation and did not require institutions to give up what they were doing—that is, the new programs were "add-ons." As important as external funds—indeed, more important—was that World War II ushered in the age of psychology or the age of mental health, manifesting itself in the larger society not only in a heightened consciousness about matters psychological but also in pressures for services that would reflect such concerns (Sarason, 1977, 1981). However, although the societal significance of these two factors cannot be overestimated, one can unjustifiably overestimate the degree to which medical school–hospital settings appropriately reflect the sea-swell alterations in societal expectations. If one agrees, as I do, with the concerns voiced today by medical educators, what requires explanation is why the level of caring and compassion among physicians, far from appropriately reflecting societal expectations, is perceived as having deteriorated. It is possible, of course, that the medical educators are vastly overstating their case. There has been no outcry on that score from the medical community. And if many in that community privately disagree with these educators, I would be surprised if any of them would assert that the problem is not a serious one.

This book is not primarily about physicians and medical education. If they have been the focus in this chapter, as they will be in the next one, it is because issues surrounding caring and compassion in the clinical endeavor have been pointedly and publicly articulated at least once each decade in regard to the medical setting. The public needs no instruction about the

role of caring and compassion in these settings, and when a minority of medical educators express their concerns about those
matters, they are addressing their professional community, not
the public. But these issues extend far beyond the medical community. The defining characteristic of the role of the clinician is
that the clinician does his or her best, on the basis of formal
training and experience, to be helpful to someone in regard to a
problem that is causing personal distress. Unfortunately, from
my perspective, we have been literally schooled to restrict the
application of the title *clinician* to professional groups who, by
tradition or by legal or professional certification or licensure,
are given the right to use the title—physicians, clinical psychologists, clinical nurses, clinical social workers, (most recently)
clinical sociologists, and clinical educators. (Not all physicians
become clinicians in the sense that they seek to help individuals
with problems.)

Indeed, in the post-World War II period, the number of
groups that has emerged presenting themselves as clinicians,
whether they use that title or not, is very large. Predictably,
their emergence has been greeted by both disdain and opposition from the more established clinical groups. That opposition
takes many forms, but certainly one of them is that the desire
to be caring, compassionate, and helpful is no warrant to assume the obligations of the clinical role. Such a desire is a
necessary but not sufficient qualification, a conclusion with
which these groups agree, but they then go on to disagree about
what is necessary and sufficient. In many of these conflicts between established and aspiring groups, the latter criticize the
former for not having a sufficiently caring and compassionate
attitude precisely because their education and training are antithetical to adopting or sustaining such an attitude. So, for
example, the public is unaware that many nursing educators
(for example, deans of prestigious nursing schools) not only
have declared their independence of physicians but also seek to
train nurses for different clinical roles in private offices and the
homes of clients. And this development rests primarily on the
argument that medical practice is too often insensitive to what
patients need and where that need is best met. For nurses, it is

an old story that in the hospital the duration of contact between physicians and patient tends to be so brief as to make a
mockery of the claim that caring and compassion characterize
the contact, frequently putting the additional burden on the
nurse to compensate for what the physician did not or could
not do. From the standpoint of what patients need once they
leave the hospital, the independent nurse, the argument goes,
has the requisite knowledge compassionately to render services
of a kind (therapeutic, preventive, informational) that no physician would. I imply, at this point, no judgment on this type of
group conflict. Its significance inheres in the agreement on both
sides that there is an intimate relation between the substance,
goals, and style of education and training, on the one hand, and
the degree to which the outlook and actions of the student reflect a caring and compassionate stance, on the other. It is recognized, of course, that, independent of education and training,
people differ markedly less in the caring and compassionate attitude and more in caring and compassionate actions. But they
both agree that what I have generally called socialization into a
profession has indisputable impact on the degree and style with
which the caring and compassionate stance appropriately informs actions. I am reminded here of the time I found myself
defending to a nurse a physician friend of mine who, the nurse
said, had acted very insensitively to a patient. "He is a very nice
guy," I said. To which the nurse replied: "I am not interested in
or affected by what is in his heart. I am by his actions."

The specific clinical groups I have mentioned direct themselves explicitly to remedying aspects of an individual's health,
and, regardless of differences of opinion about their activity, we
have no difficulty understanding why they call themselves clinicians. Each asserts that its activity derives from a body of knowledge, research, and experience that accounts for the therapeutic
value of the activity. How shall we regard lawyers? They do not
regard themselves as clinicians. But what about the lawyers who
devote themselves to helping individuals seeking a divorce, with
children frequently in the picture? The number of such lawyers
is not minuscule; and, of course, the number of such clients is
very large. Although these lawyers do not regard themselves as

clinicians, they are never in doubt that they are dealing with problems serious and fateful in their consequences for the lives of people. Like it or not, and they tend not to like it, they are quintessentially in the role of the clinician trying to understand and help someone with problems in living, problems that require, among other things, that the lawyer be caring and compassionate.

How effective are lawyers in this aspect of their helping role? How frequently do they define their role so narrowly as to justify not having to give expression to caring and compassionate feelings? If we assume without question that physicians should be caring and compassionate, and if failure to behave appropriately evokes indictments from within and without the profession, why have not our scrutiny and concern been directed toward lawyers, many of whom deal in the protected confines of their offices with individual and family misery? I shall have more to say about this later in the book. If I ask these questions here about lawyers, it is to illustrate the more general point that in the post–World War II period there has been a veritable explosion both in the number of people who seek help to reduce the agonies of personal distress (whatever its form and sources) and in the number of groups seeking to fulfill a clinical role. But the word *groups* is misleading, because there are thousands of individuals, particularly in our urban areas, who are not members of any of these groups but who offer (frequently through advertisements in daily or weekly newspapers) services to people in distress. And one must note the startling increase in the number of radio programs devoted exclusively to advice giving to people with personal problems, those giving advice frequently having no special credentials other than a caring, compassionate attitude. If one listens, as I frequently do, to these programs—in the larger New York metropolitan area, I have identified at least a dozen such programs, not counting those that are on from midnight to dawn—three of their features are relevant here.

First, there are many people "out there" who not only listen to these advice givers but also respect and even revere them for their caring and advice. Second, it is by no means in-

frequent for individuals to say that they are calling because of
dissatisfaction with the kind of caring and help they have received from professionals—physicians, lawyers, and an assort-
ment of mental health personnel. Third, the substance and
appropriateness of their advice aside, these advice givers convey
a caring and compassionate stance—they convey a willingness to
listen, understand, and be helpful—but always with the restric-
tions imposed by available time, a restriction that we shall see
later is frequently used by professionals to inhibit acting on the
basis of caring and compassionate feelings aroused in them.
Time, of course, is a limited resource, but it is one thing to rationalize the sources of its limited availability and quite another
thing to justify its consequences for clinicians and clients. This
is less a manifestation of the personality characteristics of individual clinicians and more of the pressures that are the consequences of the economic and/or organizational basis of clinical
work. But, as any medical or other kinds of clinical trainees can
attest, the time pressures that characterize their training experiences subtly and inexorably alter their personality in regard to
caring and compassionate behavior. Just as the personality of
the worker on the assembly line, where time is also such a limited resource, undergoes changes as a defense against the lack of
personal expression, so does the budding clinician change in response to the pressures of limited time, and one of these
changes has to do with the perceived need to limit the expression of caring and compassion. This is understandable, let alone
changeable, not in terms of an individual psychology but rather
in terms of the culture of the setting in which socialization into
clinical work takes place.

What is the significance in this matter of the truly amazing increase in self-help groups? There is hardly a condition of
personal and bodily distress for which a self-help group, local
and national, cannot be found. I have known many of these
groups, and there is no doubt in my mind that two of the factors accounting for their exponential increase are, first, dissatisfaction with the caring and compassion they have received from
professional clinicians and, second, the related belief that only
those who have the condition can understand what having that

condition means and, therefore, can be helpful to each other. Indeed, some of these groups will have nothing to do with professionals, and some will establish contact with professionals but restrict their roles.[3] These attitudes of criticism and disdain are sometimes directed to clinicians who understand and agree with these criticisms, who want to be helpful in some way, and who feel unjustifiably excluded. Only in the past decade have a few clinicians stimulated and helped develop self-help groups, and, in my experience, at least, they have tended to be newer entrants to their professional field, products of the sixties, when almost every profession (and every major societal institution) was indicted for its lack of caring and compassion, a direct consequence of its insensitivity to inequities in providing services. In this connection, I should note still another characteristic of self-help groups: The individuals who join these groups may or may not be critical of this or that clinician, but in some vague way they tend to be critical of a "system" of service in which, in different ways, both patient and clinician are victims.

      In this chapter, I have not attempted to analyze in detail the issues surrounding caring and compassion in the clinical endeavor. The major thrust of this chapter was the more modest one of indicating that, although the issues have been raised (again) in relation to the field of medicine, they go beyond that

---

[3] Several years ago, the federal Congress passed legislation to provide mental health services for Vietnam veterans, legislation for which these veterans had been vigorously lobbying. Although that program was administratively housed in the Veterans Administration (VA), the sites for these services around the country were never in VA hospitals or clinics; they were in the community. That was no accident, because the Vietnam veterans group made three things clear: only a Vietnam veteran could understand the experiences of another Vietnam veteran; the staff had to be Vietnam veterans, and the emphasis had to be on peer counseling. They wanted no part of any of the VA mental health professional groups, and, therefore, to avoid domination by them and accommodation to their treatment philosophy, these services could not be provided in the usual VA hospital or clinic. In their presentation on public television, the president of the Vietnam veterans group stated in the most unvarnished fashion that to expect mental health professionals to be caring and compassionate toward Vietnam veterans was to fly in the face of the experience of veterans. The stance of these veterans toward clinicians was identical to that one finds in many self-help groups.

field, and to an extent that justifies taking seriously the assumption that the clinician's behavior and the patient's perception of that behavior are interrelated expressions of more than individual and institutional factors in the sense that they are never independent of features of the larger society. And that is the point: precisely because they are never independent, and they were and are products of a society's dominant ideology and social history, efforts to influence individual and institutional practice will enjoy little success unless those efforts derive from widespread changes in the society. If caring and compassionate behavior, its frequency and quality, have come to have a problematic status in the clinical endeavor, let us not unreflectively resort to remedies that, however understandable and laudable, are not likely to pay us the dividends we seek. This, I should not have to emphasize, does not mean that you give up your efforts to improve the frequency and quality of clinicians' caring and compassionate behavior or the institutional context in which professionals are trained and go out, Don Quixote style, to make society over. How can one justify silent acquiescence in the face of an individual clinician's uncaring and uncompassionate behavior? How can one justify similar acquiescence to an institutional context that you perceive to reinforce such behavior? Morally, you have no choice in either instance but to blow the whistle, to do what you think can be done, assuming that you are in a position where blowing the whistle may stop or alter what is undesirable, however modest and transient the effects might be. But in blowing the whistle, let us recognize that if what we want to change does not reflect significant pressures from the larger society, we are lacking one of the crucial ingredients that force institutional change. This, as we shall see in the next chapter, is well illustrated by the impact on medicine of the Flexner report of 1910. If my point is well illustrated by that deservedly famous report, it also confirms the maxim that you always pay a price. And in regard to the problematic status today of caring, compassionate behavior in medical clinicians, we are still paying a price unintended by Abraham Flexner.

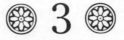

Training of Physicians:
The Unintended Impact
of the Flexner Report
on Medical Education

It is impossible to write even a semiserious history of American medicine in this century without discussing the 1910 Flexner report on *Medical Education in the United States and Canada.* Fifty years after its publication, it was reprinted (Flexner [1910], 1960), because it was considered both "a landmark in the history of medical training" and "a classic in the literature of education." Although there is no disputing these characterizations, the thrust of this chapter is that the Flexner report, a product of its times, had one serious blind spot, the unintended consequence of which was to set the stage for the cyclical emergence of concern about what medical education does to caring and compassionate behavior in physicians. If American medicine feels a deep indebtedness to Flexner and venerates his report, it is in part because it has been unable to ask what price was paid for the benefits that report brought to American medicine and the larger society.

Contrary to conventional wisdom, the Flexner report was not a revolutionary document, a fact recognized by Flexner himself. The report contained several interrelated themes. The first, and by far the most fateful in terms of educational impact, was that the time had come for medical education to be more solidly based on the fruits and traditions of science and scientific research. In this respect, the report was an unusually clear statement of an ongoing trend gaining increasing recognition and strength, best represented in several medical schools. The wedding between science and medical education, Flexner emphasized, could not take place within a two-year medical school curriculum, especially when it was possible (as it was) to enter medical school directly from high school or with a minimum of two years in a college. And that wedding, as the following words of Flexner make plain, would require changes in the undergraduate preparation of those seeking a career in medicine. For Flexner, the issues surrounding medical education would and should alter premedical education.

> The physician's concern with normal process is not disinterested curiosity; it is the starting point of his effort to comprehend and to master the abnormal. Pathology and bacteriology are the sciences concerned with abnormalities of structure and function and their causation. Now the agents and forces which invade the body to its disadvantage play their game, too, according to law. And to learn that law one goes once more to the same fundamental sciences upon which the anatomist and the physiologist have already freely drawn,—viz., biology, physics, and chemistry.
>
> Nor do these apparently recondite matters concern only the experimenting investigator, eager to convert patiently acquired knowledge of bacterial and other foes into a rational system of defense against them. For the practical outcome of such investigation is not communicable by rote; it cannot be reduced to prescriptions for mechanical use by the unenlightened practitioner. Modern medicine cannot be formulated in quiz-compends; those who would employ it must trouble to under-

stand it. Moreover, medicine is developing with
beneficient rapidity along these same biological
and chemical lines. Is our fresh young graduate of
five and twenty to keep abreast of its progress? If
so, he must, once more, understand; not otherwise
can he adopt the new agents and new methods is-
suing at intervals from each of a dozen fertile laboratories; for rote has no future; it stops where it is.
"There can be no doubt," said Huxley, "that the
future of pathology and of therapeutics, and therefore of practical medicine, depends upon the extent to which those who occupy themselves with
these subjects are trained in the methods and im-
pregnated with the fundamental truths of biology." Now the medical sciences proper—anatomy,
physiology, pathology, pharmacology—already
crowd the two years of the curriculum that can be
assigned to them; and in so doing, take for granted
the more fundamental sciences—biology, physics,
and chemistry—for which there is thus no adequate
opportunity within the medical school proper.
Only at the sacrifice of some essential part of the
medical curriculum—and for every such sacrifice
the future patients pay—can this curriculum be
made to include the preliminary subjects upon
which it presumes.

From the foregoing discussion, these conclusions emerge: By the very nature of the case, admission to a really modern medical school must at
the very least depend on a competent knowledge
of chemistry, biology, and physics. Every depar-
ture from this basis is at the expense of medical
training itself. From the exclusive standpoint of
the medical school it is immaterial where the students get the instruction. But it is clear that if it is
to become the common minimum basis of medical
education, some recognized and organized manner
of obtaining it must be devised: It cannot be left to

the initiative of the individual without greatly impairing its quality. Regular provision must therefore be made at a definite moment of normal educational progress. Now the requirement above agreed on is too extensive and too difficult to be incorporated in its entirety within the high school or to be substituted for a considerable portion of the usual high school course; besides, it demands greater maturity than the secondary school student can be credited with except towards the close of his high school career. The possibility of mastering the three sciences outside of school may be dismissed without argument. In the college or technical school alone can the work be regularly, efficiently, and surely arranged for. The requirement is therefore necessarily a college requirement, covering two years, because three laboratory courses cannot be carried through in a briefer period,—a fortunate circumstance, since it favors the student's simultaneous development along other and more general lines. It appears, then, that a policy that at the outset was considered from the narrow standpoint of the medical school alone shortly involves the abandonment of this point of view in favor of something more comprehensive. The preliminary requirement for entrance upon medical education must therefore be formulated in terms that establish a distinct relation, pedagogical and chronological, between the medical school and other educational agencies. Nothing will do more to steady and to improve the college itself than its assumption of such definite functions in respect to professional and other forms of special training [pp. 24-26].

If the call for a more science-based medical curriculum was not revolutionary, the practical implications of that call for undergraduate and high school curricula were radical. Flexner was an educator, and a very astute one, and it would have been surprising if, in focusing on medical schools, he did not pursue the implications of his observations for education in premedical years. The shaping of the scientific physician would begin long before he or she began medical school.

The second theme was still another reflection of Flexner the educator. To understand the scientific underpinnings of medical practice required at least two conditions: the medical student would be provided the conditions for *doing* science, so to speak, and be required to do it, and his mentors, his role models, would be individuals who would be devoted to research. Science, for Flexner, could not be for the medical student or his teachers abstractions divorced from doing and application.

> Investigation and practice are thus one in spirit, method, and object. What is apt to be regarded as a logical, is really but a practical, difficulty, due to the necessity for a division of labor. "The golden nuggets at or near the surface of things have been for the greater part discovered, it seems safe to say. We must dig deeper to find new ones of equal value, and we must often dig circuitously, with mere hints for guides." If, then, we differentiate investigator and practitioner, it is because in the former case action is leisurely and indirect, and in the latter case, immediate and anxious. The investigator swings around by a larger loop. But the mental qualities involved are the same. They employ the same method, the same sort of intelligence. And as they get their method and develop their intelligence in the first place at school, it follows that the modern medical school will be a productive as well as a transmitting agency. An exacting discipline cannot be imparted except in a keen atmosphere by men who are themselves "in training." Of course, the business of the medical school is the making of doctors; nine-tenths of its graduates will, as Dr. Osler holds,

never be anything else. But practitioners of modern medicine must be alert, systematic, thorough, critically open-minded; they will get no such training from perfunctory teachers. Educationally, then, research is required of the medical faculty because only research will keep the teachers in condition. A non-productive school, conceivably up to date to-day, would be out of date to-morrow; its dead atmosphere would soon breed a careless and unenlightened dogmatism [p. 56].

As for the student, Flexner states:

The student is throughout to be kept on his mettle. He does not have to be a passive learner, just because it is too early for him to be an original explorer. He can actively master and securely fix scientific technique and method in the process of acquiring the already known. From time to time a novel turn may indeed give zest to routine; but the undergraduate student of medicine will for the most part acquire the methods, standards, and habits of science by working over territory which has been traversed before, in an atmosphere freshened by the search for truth [p. 57].

It is getting ahead of the story somewhat, but in fairness to Flexner and as a corrective to the present perception of his report, I must note that he explicitly states that, although the bulk of the medical faculty would be involved in research, there should be room for a special type of teacher:

On the other hand, it will never happen that every professor in either the medical school or the university faculty is a genuinely productive scientist. There is room for men of another type,—the non-productive, assimilative teacher of wide learning, continuous receptivity, critical sense, and re-

sponsive interest. Not infrequently these men,
catholic in their sympathies, scholarly in spirit and
method, prove the purveyors and distributors
through whom new ideas are harmonized and made
current. They preserve balance and make connections. The one person for whom there is no place
in the medical school, the university, or the college, is precisely he who has hitherto generally
usurped the medical field,—the scientifically dead
practitioner, whose knowledge has long since come
to a standstill and whose lectures, composed when
he first took his chair, like pebbles rolling in a
brook get smoother and smoother as the stream of
time washes over them [p. 56].

That special, scientifically unproductive teacher would have
little chance today of receiving tenure in a medical school! Unfortunately, Flexner says no more than what is in that paragraph, which lends itself to at least two interpretations. The narrow interpretation is that Flexner, again the educator, recognizes
that there are individuals who, however scientifically unproductive themselves, keep abreast of scientific advances and have a
special talent for communicating and integrating those advances
in exciting and challenging ways. They are superb teachers. Another interpretation is that there should be room for someone
else, who, like Socrates, raises important issues and poses hard
questions whose thrust is to call into question moral, ethical, social, and educational aspects of medicine and science—for example, the problems inherent in resting medicine almost exclusively
on a narrow scientific foundation—someone who, in different ways from various perspectives, enlarges the self-conscious-
ness of colleagues and students about the means and ends of
medical education and practice. Is there a medical school today
that would seriously hire and give tenure to the likes of *Mister*
Flexner? I would like to believe, and nothing known about him
controverts it, that Abraham Flexner, an "unproductive scientist," would be astonished if he were told that there was no permanent place for him on a medical school faculty. To raise and

investigate ideas that require no laboratory, that will not alter the direction of a scientific field, but that are explicitly relevant to medicine as a social, moral, economic, political, and educational enterprise—would the performance of that role have been seen by Flexner as inimical to his conception of what belongs before the intellectual forum of the medical school community? Flexner uses the phrase "educated man" several times, and there can be no doubt that, for him, that phrase was an antonym to "provincial." More of this later.

A third theme in the report, stated in Pritchett's introduction and repeated many times in the rest of the report, is quality over quantity. More specifically, there were too many medical schools, many of which were shoddy commercial enterpises, turning out too many ill-trained physicians. If anything in the report caught the public eye, it was Flexner's observations and analysis of every existing medical school. These descriptions provided ample basis for the conclusion that many of these medical schools did not serve the public interest and did not deserve to exist. Most, but not all, of these medical schools were unconnected with universities, and their connection with a hospital was tenuous in the extreme or even nonexistent. It was a messy, scandalous situation that could no longer be tolerated. Flexner did not uncover these conditions; they were already known and discussed. In fact, a number of these kinds of schools had already begun to disappear, and some that Flexner studied were on very shaky grounds (financial and otherwise) and were seeking to be absorbed by universities. Flexner's contribution, and no mean one, inhered in his terse, objective descriptions and in his coverage of all existing medical schools. Given Flexner's credentials, the fact that the study was initiated, supported, and circulated by the Carnegie Foundation for the Advancement of Teaching, and the support he received by leading medical school educators, there was no way, so to speak, that the substance of his report could be ignored. The report was by the right person, under the right aegis, at the right time.

The recommendation to reduce the number of medical schools and physicians did not stem only from the poor quality of the existing schools. The recommendation was also a conse-

quence of the logic of Flexner's conception of what medical
education required. If the curriculum was to be enlarged and
prolonged to accommodate the range of the relevant sciences
other than in token ways, if the appropriate laboratories were
to be developed and well maintained, if the medical school was
to be productively and creatively integrated with a hospital setting, and if all of this was to be developed within the scholarly
and research traditions of the university, it was obvious that
many existing medical schools simply could not muster the
necessary intellectual and financial resources. The way in which
Flexner posed and defined the goals of medical education almost automatically meant that the number of medical schools
would decrease. Although that meant fewer physicians, it also
meant, Flexner asserted, that the dramatic improvement in the
scientific quality of medical training would more than compensate for reduction in numbers.

> The proper method of calculating cost is,
> however, social. Society defrays the expense of
> training and maintaining the medical corps. In the
> long run which imposes the greater burden on the
> community, the training of a needlessly vast body
> of inferior men, a large proportion of whom break
> down, or that of a smaller body of competent men
> who actually achieve their purpose? When to the
> direct waste here in question there is added the in-
> direct loss due to incompetency, it is clear that the
> more expensive type is decidedly the cheaper.
> Aside from interest on investment, from loss by
> withdrawal of the student body from productive
> occupations, the cost of our present system of
> medical education is annually about $3,000,000,
> as paid in tuition fees alone. The number of high-
> grade physicians really required could be educated
> for much less; the others would be profitably em-
> ployed elsewhere; and society would be still fur-
> ther enriched by efficient medical service [p. 43].

I have tried, albeit very sketchily, to present the spirit and some of the substance of Flexner's report. For the reader intrigued with how much of the present not only reflects but contains the past, the report is an eye-opener. For those (including those who either wrote or read subsequent reports on problems of medical education) endeavoring to alter in any way the direction of medical education, reading the original report is essential, if only to ponder the question: In what ways are the sources of concern today about medical education direct consequences of what the report said and did not say? Veneration of that report has been an effective obstacle to asking that question, setting the stage for further confirmation of the maxim that the more things change, the more they remain the same. But, as I indicated earlier, there are medical educators today who, insofar as the issue of caring and compassion among physicians is concerned, argue that the situation is not the same but has got worse. Could it be that for the origins of this problem we should turn to Mr. Flexner's views of the problem? Let me address that question now, for which the preceding pages of this chapter have been prologue.

Flexner says virtually nothing about caring and compassion in physicians. Indeed, except for his forceful emphasis on preparation in science as a prerequisite for entrance to medical school, he does not discuss criteria for selection. That omission, it is safe to assume, in no way reflects Flexner's insensitivity to the importance of these personal characteristics in physicians. If that omission reflects anything, it is Flexner's assumption— one of those "of course" assumptions—that, generally speaking, people who sought a career in medicine were prompted by a "calling," a term he explicitly uses almost in passing. Today, that term has an antique flavor, a remnant of a long ago when it was the rule, not the exception, to believe that one's plans and life had transcendental origins and meanings. It was not that one exercised no choice in the matter but rather that that choice had to reflect the feeling that, in a larger moral-ethical-spiritual scheme of things, one had a special place: a role that uniquely integrated one's special interests and abilities with the rendering of a service. And to be "called" meant that you took on the obligation to be governed by the rules and traditions of that larger, transcendent scheme of things. A calling presented you with an opportunity to serve; it also meant that you would be governed by a "higher" set of moral-ethical obligations, which, precisely because of their transcendental significance, meant that the needs of those one served took precedence over one's own. It was expected that "calling" would frequently require self-sacrifice.

Living as most of us do in a very secular world, in which a phrase such as "transcendental scheme of things" smacks of mysticism and superstition, it is hard for us to comprehend the concept of a "calling." But for Flexner, as for many others of his time, that was no problem. The idea that one embarked on a medical career for monetary or purely personal reasons was an idea that Flexner derogated. For example, Flexner goes to some length to invalidate the claim that reducing the number of medical schools and physicians would have untoward effects on medical services in rural areas. In the course of his argument, he says:

> What is the financial inducement that persuades men scientifically inclined to do what they really like:—for a man who does not like medicine has no business in it. How far does the investment point of view actually control? Complete and reliable data are at hand. The college professor has procured for himself an even more elaborate and expensive training than has here been advocated for the prospective physician. Did he require the assurance of large dividends on his investment? "The full professor in the one hundred institutions in the United States and Canada which are financially strongest receives on the average an annual compensation of approximately $2500." But the scholar does not usually advance beyond the assistant professorship: what figure has financial reward cut with him? "At the age of twenty-six or

twenty-seven, after seven years of collegiate and graduate study, involving not only considerable outlay, but also the important item of the foregoing of earning during this period, he is the proud possessor of his Ph.D. and is ready to enter his profession. The next five years he spends as instructor. In his thirty-second year he reaches assistant professorship. He is now in his thirty-seventh year, having been an assistant professor for five years. His average salary for the ten years has been $1325. ... At thirty-seven he is married, has one child, and a salary of $1800." In Germany "the road to a professorship involves a period of training and of self-denial far longer and more exacting than that to which the American professor submits;" in France "there are no pecuniary prizes whatever in their calling for even those who attain its highest posts." What is even more to the point,—the posts of instructor and assistant in small colleges situated in out-of-the-way places can be readily filled at slender salaries with expensively trained men. Of course there are compensations. But the point is that a large financial inducement is not indispensable, provided a man is doing what he likes. In most sections the country doctor has better worldly prospects. The fact stands out that it is not income but taste that primarily attracts men into scholarly or professional life. That granted, the prospect of a modest income does not effectually deter; and not infrequently the charm of living away from large cities may even attract [p. 44].

Flexner's conception of what should be appropriate motivations for entering a medical career was in part, and no small part, a reaction to the practice of many medical schools to entice students to their programs because they would lead to monetary rewards. In some cases, Flexner points out, the advertising budgets of these schools was larger than that for laboratories! No, for Flexner, it was morally inadequate to seek a medical career for financial gain. The physician had to have "higher," more morally demanding, less personal reasons. For Flexner, the physician's obligation to the sick and to the larger society took precedence over personal aggrandizement in any manner, shape, or form.

There are those who would argue that Flexner had an idealized image of what kind of person a physician should be, an image no more found in 1910 than among "real" physicians today. That may be the case, as I shall soon argue, but that should not obscure the fact that what exercised Flexner was the number of people who were entering medicine for the wrong reasons; that is, for narrow, personal, selfish reasons. (If Flexner's idealized physician is no more frequent today than in 1910, it is well that he is not alive today.)

In 1975, years before I read the Flexner report, I conducted a study that is relevant here. The study (Sarason, Sarason, and Cowden, 1975) was concerned with the satisfactions from work among highly educated professionals, mostly in law and medicine. What had been their expectations, and how well were they realized? The study was not concerned, methodologically or theoretically, with personality characteristics but rather with other factors bearing on career choice and its perceived satisfactions. The title of the book in which that study was further discussed was *Work, Aging, and Social Change: Professionals and the One-Life-One-Career Imperative* (Sarason, 1977). I was not then interested in such things as caring and compassionate attitudes and behavior. We interviewed college seniors, most of whom had decided on medicine or law as careers, medical and law students, and lawyers and physicians at different stages of their careers. The interviews were semistructured and allowed the interviewees opportunities to bring up and discuss anything they thought was or had been relevant to choice of career.

For starters, let me focus on the replies of the premedical students to the question: What satisfactions do you expect to experience from your career in medicine? High income, travel, high social status, and interesting work were the most frequent

answers. Travel was the single most frequent response. Not
everyone spontaneously mentioned high income, but it was obvious from follow-up questions and the total interview that high
income was a given, requiring neither mention nor elaboration.
It was one of those "of course" assumptions. These replies were
only mildly surprising to me, having spent as I had by that time
three decades in or around medical schools, some of that time
directly devoted to teaching medical students. After analyzing
the interviews and pondering their significances for career
choice and work satisfaction, it dawned on me one day that I
could not recall a single interview during which the student had
said—spontaneously or in regard to any question or discussion
in the hour or more long interview—that he or she had chosen
medicine to help people, to contribute in some selfless or idealistic way to the betterment of society, to put any form of personal aggrandizement secondary to service to others and to the
improvement of a larger scheme of things. No, I did not expect
that the bulk, or even a significant fraction, of the students
would give expression to whatever is implied in the concept of a
"calling." The absence of that expectation is noteworthy in itself. But there was a subliminal part of my thinking that did expect that some of these students, at least one or two, would
describe themselves in relation to a medical career in idealistic
terms. None had, although there had been ample opportunity
for them to do so.

If we now turn to medical students, we find the same responses to the question about expectations, but now their responses have to be seen in the context of how they experience
themselves in the medical school–hospital setting. They are ex-
quisitely aware that they are being socialized to think and act in
certain ways, their personal thinking, values, and style to the
contrary notwithstanding. They are vastly discouraged, indeed
overwhelmed, by the discrepancy between what they know and
what they should know, a discrepancy that in no way lessens as
they go from first to fourth year. For all practical purposes,
they have little time to think, reflect, raise questions, or pose
issues with their mentors, especially if what is on their minds
smacks of the philosophical. The troubling personal-ethical-

moral issues get taken up in informal discussion with other students. They view themselves as slowly but surely forced to give up what they see as their idealism in order to adapt to another ever-increasing discrepancy: the gulf between what pressured time allows them to give in an interpersonal sense to patients and what these patients need and want. The consequences of that discrepancy are exacerbated by a feeling of discomfort, even incompetence, about their ability to deal with many of their sick, anxious, and (to them) interpersonally difficult patients. But as one fourth-year student said: "If we had to deal with the psychological, the situation would be worse, because we would not know how to do it well. Keep a distance, play it cool, and deal with their illness. That's what we see our professors do." Finally, and with startling clarity, these students report that they are presented with a choice: Do I want to be a first-class citizen in the medical community by devoting myself to research and science, or do I want to be a second-class citizen by virtue of becoming *just* a practitioner? If the medical student (the situation is no different in the residency years) learns anything, it is that, although the private practitioner serves a useful role, it is far less worthy than that of the medical scientist. In the ideology that powers the medical school, the faculty is analogous to the College of Cardinals, and the community practitioners are the priests, with no bishops as intermediaries. For many medical students, this scale of values plays into and exacerbates feelings of unworthiness and deficit stemming from other sources.

There are many significances that one could derive from what premedical students reported. For my present purpose, I venture the opinion that neither do medical schools select students by criteria appropriate to Flexner's implicit conception of who should enter medicine nor does the atmosphere or the curriculum of these schools engender and reinforce caring and compassionate behavior. I should remind the reader that it is the concern today of medical educators about the lack or weakness of caring and compassionate behavior in physicians that suggested to me that I should do what few people today do: read the original Flexner report. What light does that report shed on current concerns? That reading very clearly indicates that Flexner concluded not only that the substance of the medical curriculum was generally scandalously inadequate but that the lack of standards and the enticements of financial gain attracted the wrong people with the wrong motivations for a medical career. Implicit in the report is a picture of the physician dedicated to a calling, a role that required adherence to a code of values and performance that transcended narrow personal and material considerations; indeed, a code that was a form of control against people's proclivity for self-aggrandizement in any of its forms. Flexner's picture of the scientist dedicated selflessly to the pursuit of knowledge and truth was matched by the picture of a person selflessly dedicated to others *and* to the betterment of the larger society. Flexner was as much the moralist as he was the educator. He would, I think it fair to say, be aghast at the concern today of medical educators about the superficiality of caring and compassion among physicians.

That brings us to the major blind spot in Flexner's report, a consequence of his exclusive, indeed obsessive, concern with scientific training—its direct impact on selection of students, its control over the curriculum—and his complete inability to consider the unintended negative consequences of his recommendations. In the realm of human affairs, there are always unintended consequences. It is one thing to force oneself to recognize that brute fact and to try, albeit always imperfectly, to get some sense of the realm of unintended consequences. It is another thing to proceed as if we live in a world where one's intended consequences will be the only consequence. Illusions are governed by our wishes, and nowhere is this better illustrated than by the frequency with which we restrict our thinking to intended consequences. This is said not as criticism of Flexner, let alone as blame, but as recognition of the fact that Flexner was quite human.

In terms of the medical curriculum, Flexner was faced with the practical problem of what could reasonably be included in four years of medical school. It seems clear that from the outset he had concluded that a scientifically based medical education could not be achieved within those four years unless those foundations began to be built in the undergraduate years and, in addition, there were postgraduate opportunities for keeping up to date on scientific and technological advances. Sophisticated curriculum developer that he was, Flexner knew that time was a most precious commodity, to be apportioned in ways that did not do violence to either the letter or the spirit of the goals of integrating science and medical practice. The basic medical sciences, as Flexner conceived them, were to be assimilated not as arid, isolated bodies of knowledge but in relation to a stepwise series of exposures to clinical phenomena and practice. Every step of the game was to serve the purpose of deepening the integration between knowledge and application. Flexner was not out to train technicians of limited knowledge and skills who dispensed their wares in uncritical, even mindless kinds of ways. That, of course, was the kind of physician he saw the bulk of medical schools to be producing. Flexner's aim was to forge a new kind of professional, steeped in and dedicated to science and its application to medical practice. That would take time and a special kind of educational ambience in which this new kind of physician would be nurtured.

Flexner did not assume that this integration would take place by itself or by a social osmosis or by the consequences of the right intentions. It could take place only if that integration was the central focus of student and faculty, not only informing what goes on but also justifying vigilance and efforts at improvement.

Flexner never asked these questions: How do we ensure that the medical student becomes a caring and compassionate physician? By what educational procedures do we instill and judge a student's understanding not only of a person's symptoms and bodily condition but of that person's experienced plight? If we seek to engender in the student a scientific conscience by which the student and we will judge action, what should be the substance of that other conscience that tells us what we "owe" others in our interpersonal, social commerce with them? Are there values or considerations that justify restricting the scope of the effort to recognizing and diluting the personal and familial anxiety, pain, and misery accompanying physical illness? Are the symptoms of these accompaniments—their prevention as well as dilution—less important than symptoms of bodily malfunction? Can we arrange a productive wedding between science and medicine without a destructive divorce between medicine and the caring, compassionate stance and action?

If Flexner did not ask these questions, it is because he was making at least two "of course" assumptions. The first was that those who would be attracted to the new medicine would be selflessly dedicated, interpersonally sensitive people prepared to deal with all aspects of the pain and misery of illness. The physician was not only to be a scientist in the narrowest sense; he was to be someone with "insight and sympathy." Let us listen to Flexner:

> So far we have spoken explicitly of the fundamental sciences only. They furnish, indeed, the essential instrumental basis of medical education. But the instrumental minimum can hardly serve as the permanent professional minimum. It is even instrumentally inadequate. The practitioner deals with facts of two categories. Chemistry, physics, biology enable him to apprehend one set; he needs a different apperceptive and appreciative apparatus to deal with other, more subtle elements. Specific preparation is in this direction much more difficult; one must rely for the requisite insight and sympathy on a varied and enlarging cultural experience. Such enlargement of the physician's horizon is otherwise important, for scientific progress has greatly modified his ethical responsibility. His relation was formerly to his patient—at most to his patient's family; and it was almost altogether remedial. The patient had something the matter with him; the doctor was called in to cure it. Payment of a fee ended the transaction. But the physician's function is fast becoming social and preventive, rather than individual and curative. Upon him soci-

ety relies to ascertain, and through measures essentially educational to enforce, the conditions that
prevent disease and make positively for physician
and moral well-being. It goes without saying that
this type of doctor is first of all an educated man
[p. 26].

And by "an educated man," Flexner meant someone steeped in
the humanities: those traditions and bodies of knowledge concerned with the nature and vicissitudes of people's moral and
ethical relationships to each other, what humans "owed" to
fellow humans, the "shoulds and oughts" that have liberated
humanity from superstition, selfishness, and tyranny. It is to
Flexner's everlasting credit that he saw that the sciences basic to
medicine were an inadequate instrumental minimum for the
education of the complete physician.

The second "of course" assumption Flexner made was
that the medical student would be constantly and vigilantly
guided by teachers who themselves were "educated men."
These teachers would themselves be more than scientists, ever
alert to the dangers of a narrow technical training. In fact, Flexner points out that the medical student, unlike the engineering
student, "handles at one and the same time elements belonging
to vastly different categories: physical, biological, psychological
elements are involved in each other" (p. 23). It would be the
prime responsibility of the teacher to ensure that these categories would be integrated. The medical school professor would
be the exemplar of the complete physician, not of the narrow
scientist.

In short, if Flexner did not pursue certain questions, it is
not because he deemed them unimportant. *On the contrary, he
deemed them the most important questions.* If he did not pursue them, it is because he assumed they would be answered in
three ways: a broad undergraduate education, a self-selection
factor that would "call" to medicine individuals with the appropriate vision and motivation, and a medical school ambience
that exposed the student to teachers who approximated the
ideal of the scientific, caring, compassionate, socially responsi-

ble physician. How else can one explain his proposing a medical school curriculum that from beginning to end concentrated on what Flexner himself considered to be "inadequate instrumentally" as a basis for medical education? The quotation earlier that ended with Flexner's "educated man" appears on page 26 of the report. The rest of the report contains nothing relevant to the contents of that stirring paragraph.

What evidence did Flexner have for the validity of his "of course" assumptions? The fact is that the evidence—spread throughout his report—lent little or no credence to these assumptions: the great majority of medical schools lacked the appropriate ambience; those who entered these medical schools generally had the wrong motivations; and most medical students had far from the undergraduate education on which Flexner pinned his hopes. There were a few medical schools that Flexner considered as models of what he was proposing. He refers to Johns Hopkins in terms of reverence. But a close reading of the report suggests that this handful or so of medical schools met Flexner's approval because of the way they based their curriculum on the basic sciences, not because he had any evidence that they attracted, selected, and educated the type of student who approximated Flexner's ideal physician.

I am not being critical of Flexner. When one considers the year the study was done, the sorry state of medical education, the partial and often complete lack of relation between medical schools and universities and between medical schools and hospitals, the slowness with which advances in science and technology were filtering into medical training, the commercialization of medical education, how frequent it was for the medical student to have only two years or less (and sometimes none) of college—Flexner's report is deserving of praise and not criticism. But it is not criticism to say that Flexner, like us, was possessed by a world view resting on axioms that are unarticulated precisely because they seem so natural, right, and proper. The process by which we are socialized into society is one by which we assimilate axioms requiring no articulation. They are self-evidently "right." They are silent but bedrock to our view of what the world is and should be. These axioms do not become blind spots (that is, they are not recognized as such) until events in the larger society force us to challenge what was heretofore unchallengeable.

Flexner lived at a time when science as salvation, science as *the* force for human progress, science as the universal solvent for human misery, had become an unarticulated part of the world view of "educated man." This axiom did not permit Flexner to inquire into possible unintended negative consequences of a medical school curriculum that from beginning to end riveted on science and technology, that, indeed, even required suffusing the undergraduate curriculum with the same ambience.[1] The assumption that his dramatic proposals would not alter the characteristics of those who would self-select themselves for a career in medicine, that somehow or other caring, compassionate, selfless behavior (in contrast to caring, compassionate, selfless rhetoric) would not be in conflict with assimilating the substance of the new curriculum, that such behavior would be both engendered and reinforced by the student's mentors—these assumptions Flexner was unable to state and, therefore, examine or challenge. By definition, unintended consequences are not predictable. But it is one thing to propose policies completely insensitive to the fact of the inevitability of unintended consequences and quite another thing to be aware of that fact and deliberately to try to fathom what some of these unintended consequences might be, even though one knows that such fathoming will at best be very incomplete. If the road to hell is paved with good intentions, a major ingredient in the

---

[1] There is no abstract reason why training for scientific thinking and research should be in conflict with or undermine the capacity for caring and compassionate behavior; in principle the scientific physician can meet the most elevated standards for such behavior. That the scientific-technological emphasis in medical schools so frequently washes out, overwhelms, or derogates such behavior says nothing about science and volumes about the weight of traditions, moral denseness, institutional narrowness and rigidity, and (most ironic of all) an inability to articulate, scrutinize, *and* test axioms that may be myths. The failure to test cherished assumptions is a gross violation of the scientific outlook in which we must never confuse assumption with fact or passionate belief with conclusions derived from empirical test.

pavement are the unintended consequences to which one's passions and do-good tendencies precluded awareness. By and large, the professional views the do-gooder as someone who vastly oversimplifies the realities with which their proposals must deal, unaware of the myriad negative ripple effects the proposals could have. In that sense, one has to say that Flexner was the typical do-gooder. Yes, and paradoxically, he was a very sophisticated do-gooder; but to the extent that he could see medical education only as an onward and upward course on which there were no potholes about which one had to worry, Flexner was a do-gooder. He lived at a time when the "educated man" had yet to learn about potholes.

If Flexner can be faulted for anything, it is his failure to take seriously something that he notes and indicts: the commercialization of medicine. His indictment is of the many medical schools of the day that were explicitly in business to make money and of those individuals attracted to it for the same reason. That we are a capitalist society—a characterization I do not use pejoratively—in which in countless ways the desire for individual material gain, indeed aggrandizement, is stimulated and reinforced, in which success is too often equated with what Veblen termed conspicuous consumption, in which striving for upward social mobility is a socially accepted goal is a fact the implications of which Flexner did not confront. Possessed as he was by the concept of the "educated man," which in his day referred to a relatively small elite in terms of socioeconomic status, Flexner assumed that such individuals were somehow devoid of the seamy aspects of the motivation for pecuniary gain. Similarly, if his indictment did not refer to the relatively few medical schools of which he approved, it was again because he assumed that, populated as they were by educated men and by medical students with the appropriate college education, economic considerations were not important in terms either of individual motivation or of institutional organization. On this score, it is interesting and important to note that, a year before the Flexner report was published, Veblen ([1918] 1957), coming from a very different socioeconomic background, finished his book *The Higher Learning in America*. It is a book that presents a very different and less sanguine picture of the college and university as a sanctuary from the marketplace. Indeed, Veblen's penetrating analysis was far more realistic and prodromal than what is said or implied by Flexner about the onward and upward course of medical education in the university. For Veblen, unlike Flexner, the university had to reflect the dominant characteristics of the society, negative and positive.

Veblen, I think it fair to say, would not have been surprised by later reports of medical educators expressing concern about the decreasing manifestations of caring and compassion in the behavior of physicians. Flexner would have been, I believe, both surprised and upset, if only because subsequent developments invalidated his assumption that the undergraduate and graduate curricula he proposed would, by the processes of selection and self-selection as well as by the example of exemplary mentors, foster caring and compassionate behavior.

Flexner had a very narrow conception of how the nature of the society inevitably got reflected in the institutions it spawned. He had a very clear and inspiring conception of the kind of physician the society needed. And he had a clear conception of how the abstraction we call science—its truth-seeking and moral traditions—should be assimilated into the outlook and practices of physicians. However, to his everlasting credit, Flexner understood, as his words plainly convey, that, although these scientific underpinnings were necessary, they were far from sufficient. There were other "more subtle elements" even more important. But, in regard to these elements, "specific preparation is in this direction much more difficult, one must rely for the requisite insight and sympathy on a varied and enlarging cultural experience." Why is that preparation much more difficult? What does Flexner want us to understand by "varied and enlarging cultural experiences"? Why is he here so vague and general about elements that he considers the most important of all, while he is so concrete and detailed about scientific training? If the preparation of these elements is so important and much "more difficult," how does one justify reliance on something as vague and inkblottish as "varied and enlarging cultural experiences"? Flexner "solved" the problem essentially by ignoring it, by resorting uncharacteristically (for him) to expressions of hope and of unalloyed optimism about the benefits of formal education. What Flexner glossed over, together with his science-filled curriculum and his narrow conception of the kind of society he lived in (and we continue to live in), set the stage for those subsequent cyclical reports bemoaning the dilution of caring and compassionate behavior among medical students and physicians generally.

What if Flexner had not glossed over the problem? What might he have recommended? Given the development of medical education so heavily influenced by Flexner's report, what can we do to repair somewhat the "much more difficult problem" that seems to have become as troubling as it has been intractable to efforts at repair? And by *troubling*, I mean troubling not only to medical educators and to the society generally but to the community of physicians as well. If my experience is any guide, many physicians are painfully and guiltily aware that their medical education, far from engendering and reinforcing caring and compassionate behavior, interacting as that does with the economics of practice, has chilled their warmer sentiments and has produced a chasm between what they are and what they would like to be, between what they know how to give and what their patients want them to give.

I postpone to a later chapter the "what to do" kinds of issues. My major aim in this chapter has been to indicate that there is no focus in the medical curriculum on how students are aided to understand the nature, expression, and problematic aspects of the concepts of caring and compassion and to acquire the interactional skills of expression that begin to meet the criteria for caring and compassionate behavior. What I would like to do in the next chapter is to illustrate the identical situation in an arena of action that on the surface at least, is very far removed from the medical one. What does the preparation of schoolteachers have in common with the education of physicians? As we shall see, they have much in common, in terms of what their training ignores and, therefore, of the adverse consequences that such ignoring brings about.

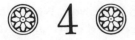

4

Inadequacies
in the Training
of Teachers and Lawyers

A clinician is someone who does the best he or she can, on the basis of formal training and experience, to help someone who comes with a problem. When the term is defined so narrowly, the distinguishing characteristic is that a problem must already exist—that is, the task is one of repair and not prevention, although the prevention of secondary and tertiary consequences of the problem is or should be always in the picture. One hopes or expects that by training and experience the clinician has been sensitized to features of an individual's appearance or behavior or self-report that suggest actions that could prevent certain problems from ever becoming manifest—that is, primary prevention. So, although the usual definition emphasizes existence of and coping with a problem, it in no way relieves the clinician from being preventer as well as repairer. Unfortunately, the training of clinicians tends to be so riveted on understanding and dealing with problems that the possibilities of prevention receive short shrift. As we saw in the previous chapter, Flexner envisioned the medical clinician both as repairer and preventer, but his emphasis was on the repair side, and he says next to nothing about the clinician as preventer. The consequences of this emphasis aside, there is another factor that contributes to avoiding or ignoring actions geared to prevention. That factor is illustrated in the joke about the patient who did not feel well and visited his physician. It was midwinter. The physician examined him and then recommended that he go home, completely undress himself, open up all the windows in his house, stand in front of a window, and breathe deeply for half an hour. The patient looked at the physician with staring disbelief and said: "But, doctor, if I do that I'll get pneumonia." To which the physician replied: "*That* I know what to do about."

Understandably, clinicians are more comfortable dealing with problems that are familiar and for which they can draw upon a course of action. The preventive stance, however, poses dilemmas to the problem-riveted, problem-trained clinician. The first is less a dilemma than it is the inability of the clinician to recognize that the patient has characteristics that may or may not be related to the presenting problem but that, if unattended to, may subsequently lead to some kind of dysfunction. For example, the individual may have a cold virus and be grossly overweight, or appear to be unaccountably "nervous," or have breath reeking of smoking, or say his or her teenager has just entered a drug abuse program—or all of these. Although one part of the clinician may know that any of these features can produce dysfunctional conditions in the individual, it does not follow that the clinician will be aware of these features or, if aware, give them the importance they deserve. What is a dilemma to the clinician, assuming that he or she recognizes the possible implications of any of these features, is whether to deal with them in light of the fact that the patient came to get help for a virus and not for reasons of life-style.

In "real life," this dilemma is exponentially exacerbated by the clinician's pervasive insecurity about, first, how to open this Pandora's box and, second, how to deal with its contents. There is little or nothing in the medical clinician's education and training that prepares him or her for dealing with (in Flexner's words) "insight and sympathy" with issues of life-style; that is, with how these issues produce problems. But, as a physician said to me: "It is not an issue of insight and sympathy. I have loads of that. I simply don't know how to be helpful in these matters. I'm not a psychologist, or psychiatrist, or social worker. I know how to be helpful about the problems my patients bring to me. Of course, they have a lot of other problems that I see that they don't talk about or want to talk about or even recognize and that will pathologically erupt down the road. But I have neither the expertise nor the time to deal effectively with them. Besides, do not underestimate how resistant patients are to hearing that they are not paying attention to something that will cause them grief in the future." What this physician was saying was that the preventive stance required understanding and actions for which his problem-oriented training did not prepare him, for which his technical, diagnostic, and treatment-repair knowledge and skills were inadequate. He was saying not that the clinical and preventive stances were conceptually or logically unrelated or in conflict but rather that he was much more comfortable with one stance than the other, that he liked to deal with issues about which he could *do* something, and that this kind of "doing" did not encompass the "doing" explicit in the preventive stance.

If the adjective *clinical* is customarily narrowly defined and conjures up images of a clinic, a hospital, physicians, and other health professionals, it has the effect of obscuring the fact that there are segments of many professions, seemingly far removed from those concerned with health, whose roles are quintessentially clinical in that they deal with the problems of individuals, problems requiring special knowledge, "insight and sympathy," and interpersonal skills geared to remediation and secondary and primary prevention. In some instances, sensitivity to the difficulties inherent in coping with already existing problems is the basis for emphasizing primary prevention. Nowhere is this emphasis more clear than in the classroom, where every teacher seeks to prevent the emergence of problems at the same time that he or she endeavors to help some students overcome an already existing problem. Indeed, one of the most frequent complaints of teachers is that they spend so much time "diagnosing and treating" problem students that it interferes with the process of teaching, intended, among other things, to prevent problems. *Clinical teaching* and *clinical supervision* are terms that have gained currency in the post-World War II era (for example, Goldhammer, 1969), testimony to the recognition that the teacher, like it or not, is a clinician dealing with problems fateful to the lives of students. One could well argue that, unlike many medical problems, which do not have percolating effects on the present and personal-social life of the individual, educational problems are rarely so encapsulated that they do not invade the student's conception of self, family, peer relationships, and future perspective. Just as the term *medical problem* too often restricts awareness of and attention to the present and future consequences of the condition, the term *educational problem* tends to convey too narrow a conception of how in the developing child a problem can suffuse major areas of functioning.

As in the case of medicine, education has again become an item high on the national agenda. Within the past few years, we have been treated to a spate of reports highly critical of schools. The criticisms are many, the tone is hortatory. These reports share one characteristic: they describe schools as if they do not contain a large number of students with major problems that impede whatever one considers normal educational development. To anyone who is familiar with our schools, especially our urban ones, these reports describe an unfamiliar world. So, for example, these reports ignore the fact and the consequences of the passage of Public Law 94-142 (the Education of Handicapped Children's Act), enacted in 1975 and intended to influence practices in every school. The definition of handicap is very general and was meant to encompass very heterogeneous conditions. But if that legislation was applicable to far more than a minuscule number of children, it did not extend to an even larger number of children who present problems to the classroom teacher.

The point is that these reports are amazingly aclinical in the degree to which they gloss over the fact that the teacher is always in the position of having to "diagnose and treat" children with obvious and significant problems. As countless teachers have said to me: "It would be nice if I could just *teach*, period. But I am expected to be a psychologist, social worker, policeman, and sometimes a substitute parent." This is like the physician who is poignantly aware that a patient has serious problems other than the one presented to him or her. But, unlike the physician, the isolated teacher in the encapsulated classroom rarely can avoid dealing with the problems surrounding a narrowly defined educational problem. Indeed, whereas we expect the physician to address a patient's specific problem—and in an era of increasing specialization, the problem becomes increasingly narrowly defined—we expect the teacher to deal with the "whole child." In this respect, we expect more of teachers than we do of any other profession. And implicit in this expectation is the assumption that the teacher is a caring and compassionate person prepared by temperament, background, and training to comprehend and appropriately react to the child's experience of his or her situation. I should emphasize that this assumption is independent of whether the teacher's diagnosis and actions are correct and appropriate. Being caring and compassionate is no guarantee that one's understanding is valid or that one's behavior is either appropriate or effective. But the expectation is that it is second nature to the teacher both to grasp and to respond to the child's experience of self, the situation, and his or her problem. When we say that the teacher starts with where the child is, we mean that the teacher almost automatically differentiates between the nature of the child's experience and that of the teacher, a differentiation as crucial as it is difficult in practice to make and sustain.

It is beyond the scope of this chapter to examine the myriad ways and times that caring and compassion are required of the teacher and to illustrate the baleful consequences of not meeting that requirement. Suffice it to say that examination is long overdue, and current critiques of our schools in general and teachers in particular deal with the problem by utterly ignoring it or, as in the case of medical education, making token gestures in regard to it. In the rest of this chapter, I restrict myself to two aspects of the issue with which most readers will be familiar, because they either are aware of the nature of our society or are parents or both.

It required no special knowledge or wisdom to predict in

1954 that one of the consequences of the Supreme Court's desegregation decision would be a dramatic sharpening in focus on
the ability of school personnel, especially teachers, to comprehend black children with whom they had had little or no classroom contact. That racial prejudice suffused the larger society
was a given, but the teacher, prejudiced or not, would, unlike
other people, be faced directly with the task of understanding
children whose experience of themselves and their world would
differ from that of other children. And that difference, if not
understood and appropriately acted on, could have adverse effects, educational and otherwise.

This problem was new only in the sense that black children were those to be understood by the teacher. It was a very
old problem in the sense that, for more than a century, teachers
had dealt with the children of the waves of immigrants whose
cultural background differed dramatically from that of teachers. Indeed, anyone familiar with the history of American education well knew that the ability *and* willingness of teachers to
try to understand these children on their own terms had been
quite poor, if not nonexistent. It was not that teachers were
cruel, insensitive people governed exclusively by mindless religious and ethnic prejudice. They were prejudiced, of course, but
it was a prejudice based, among other things, on the assumption
that immigrant parents wanted their children to be American-
ized in the ways their teachers envisioned. That assumption was
grossly incorrect. It was not that teachers were devoid of the desire to understand but rather that they could not see that their
stance of cultural superiority short-circuited the process of
understanding people who were different from themselves. Caring and compassion are virtually impossible when that process
of understanding does not take place. And those were times,
like today, when the students presented many problems that required caring and compassionate actions on the part of teachers,
not just verbalized attitudes. Already in the nineteenth century,
educational philosophers had sensitized teachers to the importance of understanding the world of the child and taking that
understanding into account in the pedagogy. But that was a sensitization to the child in the abstract, not to the varieties of im-

migrant children that teachers had in their classrooms. It was a sensitization to the child, *not* to the culturally determined stance of the teacher and to the obstacles that were presented to the teacher.

Let us bear in mind that if such sensitization was lacking among classroom teachers, it was also conspicuously absent from the understanding and actions of those in the nascent field of anthropology, in which the description of cultural differences was a central concern. This lack is understandable if we like to believe that the hindsight we have achieved from the past century and more about how cultural prejudice insidiously affects caring and compassion has dramatically altered our actions. On the level of abstract knowledge, one cannot deny that such an alteration has been achieved, but, as Gladwin (1980) poignantly and compellingly describes in the case of anthropology, on the level of action, we have no reason to be enthusiastic about how far we have come from the nineteenth century. The very concept of the "Third World" should be sufficient to remind us that an old problem has taken on a new guise.

On what basis should one have expected that teachers in the post–World War II era would have absorbed the lessons of the previous century, would have been better prepared to deal with the consequences of the 1954 desegregation decision? Unfortunately, the answer to that question is exactly the same as that to the question of how well physicians are prepared to deal caringly and compassionately with their patients. And that answer is that there was little or nothing in the preparation of teachers that would enable them to understand and appropriately respond to the world of children (and parents) different from that of teachers. As in the case of medical education, the preparation of teachers unreflectively rested on the assumption that "of course" the process of selection and self-selection for teaching ensured that teachers would be caring and compassionate people. And again, as in the case of medical education, there was the additional assumption that the mentors of teachers would be models of caring and compassionate teaching. That assumption was a blatant myth, because the mentors of teachers were never observed in the role of the schoolteacher; that is, they were members of a college faculty, not teachers in a public school classroom. It is true that for a period of weeks the students would do practice teaching in a public school, but, as any student will relate, those are weeks taken up with matters and duties that exclude any serious focus on issues of caring and compassion. And there is an additional assumption: when the student becomes a "real teacher" in a school, he or she is in a setting that stimulates, reinforces, and maximizes caring and compassionate behavior. That assumption may be a bit more valid than the assumption that the modern hospital is conducive to caring and compassionate behavior in medical personnel.

There was every reason to expect that the 1954 desegregation decision would bring to the fore long-standing issues centering around the ability of teachers to seek to understand black children and their parents other than from an unrealistically narrow conception of the process of education. It is in no way to indulge in scapegoating to say that there was every reason to expect that teachers would show no more and no less understanding of black children than their predecessors had shown earlier for immigrant children and their parents. Indeed, one had to expect less understanding because of the history of slavery in this country and all that connotes about race relations. Let us remember that, although the society had not denied immigrant children access to the schools—some have argued that for nonaltruistic reasons it was in the best interests of the society to educate them—such a denial essentially characterized society's attitude and action toward black children. The "separate but equal" doctrine ensured a quality of education for blacks far below that of immigrant children. You have only to see how blacks were depicted in movies (for example, Stepin Fetchit) and radio (for example, Amos and Andy) to begin to fathom the difference between caring and compassion, on the one hand, and derisive paternalism, on the other hand. Until relatively recently, physicians related to patients with the attitude "doctor knows best," implicit in which was the assumption of paternalism; that is, the patient was too ignorant or too emotional to be entrusted with knowledge and to participate in decisions vital to the patient's present and future status. "The less they know, the better off they are" was not an uncommon statement by physicians. Similarly, educators, reflecting the larger society, viewed blacks paternalistically. The analogy can be extended further, because, just as many patients have long had strongly ambivalent love-hate feelings toward physicians who placed them in the role of the dependent, impatient child, blacks have had similar feelings toward uncomprehending paternalistic-maternalistic teachers.

It is laboring the obvious to say that, before the desegregation decision, teachers had to deal with children who had difficult problems and that, after that decision, the number of such children increased. But if that is obvious, it is also misleading about the obligations implicit in the clinical role. More correctly, perhaps, it requires that we re-examine the definition of the clinician as someone who does the best he or she can, on the basis of experience and formal training, to help someone who comes with a problem. (Let us leave aside the fact that children very rarely come to a teacher with a problem; it is the teacher who makes the diagnosis that the child has a problem.) That definition conveys the impression that the clinician studies the individual, decides what the nature of the problem is, and then acts in ways likely to dilute or eliminate the problem. This impression is misleading to the extent that it glosses over the obligation of the clinician to take seriously the knowledge that the clinician's world is not that of the troubled individual and that the clinician must exercise control over the tendency to project the values of his or her world onto the individual. In other words, the clinician not only seeks to get into the world of the individual but also experiences a change reflected in action. The clinical role is aimed at changing something about the individual, but it is preceded by a process of change in the clinician's understanding. When that process is absent, it results in routinized, ritualistic actions that ensure a gulf between the worlds of the clinician and the individual. That process may be absent for reasons of prejudice, laziness, or inadequate training. (As we shall see in a later chapter, it may be because of age differences; for example, a young clinician with an aged patient.) In any event, if we have learned anything about the clinical role, it is the importance of exercising control over the unreflective tendency to assume an identity between the world of the clinician and that of the troubled individual. To seek to understand requires the clinician to confront obstacles within him- or herself. If, at best, we fall short of the mark, it is testimony to the importance of the effort. The clinician is always part of both the problem and the solution.

We are used to hearing that we are a pluralistic society, one that bears and will continue to bear the stamp of waves of immigration. If we needed any reminding on that score, the 1954 desegregation decision took care of that. Here, too, teachers and schools, as in the case of past waves of immigration, had to deal directly with the consequences. From the standpoint of teachers, they would now have to deal with many children, black and white, who would present them with problems in the classroom. From the standpoint of teachers, these "problems" were *in* the children. What teachers did not grasp, what their training did not prepare them to understand, was that the problem was in them as much as it was in students. That is to say, the problem of the teacher was how to understand how problem behavior in the child was embedded in and reflected a phenomenology that was distinctively individual, social, cultural, and racial in nature—unless, of course, such understanding is considered irrelevant to the effectiveness of a teacher's actions. The black child who has trouble learning to read, or who appears unmotivated, or who is destructive, or who is sassy—are these "problems" understandable only in terms of an individual psychology? Is any individual comprehensible by such a psychology? It required no special psychological sophistication in 1954 to predict that teachers would experience every insidious consequence of a narrow, individual psychology.

The "clinical issue" that needs to be raised is conceptually independent of prejudice. One may have little or no prejudice and yet be unable to undertake that process of understanding that makes the experience of caring and compassion both possible and a shaper of action. Prejudice is inimical to the clinical stance and action, but the absence of prejudice in no way guarantees that the person who finds him- or herself in a clinical role will discharge that role in appropriate ways. As I said earlier, long before the desegregation decision, teachers were in a clinical role with children (not only with children of immigrants), but there is no evidence whatsoever that, on balance, they performed well in that role. It would be surprising if it had been otherwise, because there has been (and still is) nothing in the selection and preparation of teachers that sensitizes them to and refines their grasp of the obligations and dilemmas of the clinical role. As we saw in the case of medical education, the physician is trained and socialized to take a very narrow view of the clinical role, but in the case of teachers, they are presented not with a narrow view but essentially with no view at all. In 1962, some colleagues and I wrote a book entitled *The Preparation of Teachers: An Unstudied Problem in Education* (Sarason, Davidson, and Blatt, 1960). The major theme of that book was that the training of teachers ill prepared them for the realities in the classroom; that is, what was going unstudied was the relevance of their preparation to the kinds of problems that they had to understand and manage. The relevance was slight, as many studies of teachers have demonstrated. Teachers disagree among themselves on many matters, but not on how poorly prepared they are for the "real" classroom. Like physicians who are uneasy with the knowledge that they do not know how to cope with the social and psychological matrix within which the presenting symptoms are embedded, the teacher is no less at sea when faced with children who challenge his or her understanding, patience, and capacity for caring and compassion.

Why is it so difficult to recognize that teachers cannot avoid the clinical role? Why is the preparation of teachers so irrelevant to what they later encounter and from which (like physicians) they insulate themselves? There are many parts to an answer, and I wish to mention only two of them. The first inheres in our image of a teacher: someone standing in front of a group of children imparting knowledge, asking questions, answering questions, demonstrating skills the students are expected to emulate. It is imagery that is strangely impersonal in that the teacher relates not to individuals but to a group (the whole classroom or a part of it). It is not the imagery conjured up by the adjective *clinical*—two people, one of whom seeks or needs help and the other striving to be compassionate and helpful. Now we know—certainly teachers know—that, although the usual imagery is far from unrepresentative of what would be observed in classrooms, what upsets teachers, what forces them to depart from the teacher-group structure, are students whose behavior, for one or another reason, requires that the teacher respond on a one-to-one basis. It may be one student; it frequently is more. They are the students who catapult the teacher into the clinical role, who can arouse the ire of the teacher precisely because the teacher-group structure must be changed, briefly or otherwise. Just as the physician gets annoyed when a patient asks questions or raises issues that do not allow the physician to proceed in his or her accustomed ways, so does the teacher get annoyed when student behavior requires him or her to depart from the usual structure. And yet, despite these classroom realities, the preparation of teachers continues to be governed by imagery demonstrably, in part at least, unrealistic and ultimately disillusioning to the teacher.

Let us not forget that the courses a student takes are not taught by classroom teachers, nor are they taught in meaningful relation to a "real" classroom in a school. In most teacher preparation programs, courses are usually taught by faculty who either have never taught in a public school or taught in one many years earlier. It is no secret that, in our schools of education (epsecially in the more prestigious ones), the supervision of student teaching is, on the part of the faculty, far less valued a role than research and scholarship. I do not hold to the position that not having been a classroom teacher, or not being meaningfully related to the school classroom, precludes one from being helpful to the student teacher or to a certified teacher. Nor do I believe that because you are an experienced classroom teacher, even a very good one, your credentials to supervise student teachers are automatically established. Clinically oriented supervision requires far more than factual knowledge and technique. It is quintessentially a relationship between a helper and a helpee in which the former seeks to comprehend the latter's way of thinking and approaching specific individuals in concrete situations, to suggest a rationale that puts the helpee's thinking and acting in a new perspective and suggests alternative actions, and to observe and discuss how the helpee follows through on the supervisory interaction—an ongoing give, take, and act relationship. It is a relationship in which both helper and helpee are learning about and from each other for the explicit purpose of being as helpful as possible to the third party: the individual with a problem.

The supervisory relationship is itself a clinical one, oriented as it should be to the remediation and prevention of problem-producing behavior in both the helpee and the pupil. If clinical supervision is time consuming, it is because of its importance, goals, and responsibilities.[1] If it is also a difficult task and not compatible with all temperaments, and by no means highly correlated with one's experience and proficiency as an individual clinician, it should occasion no surprise. And, I must emphasize, if clinical supervision takes place in a setting in which it is a devalued responsibility, then caring and compassionate behavior toward helpee and "patient" becomes a very chancy affair.

In medicine, the general practitioner has much less status than the specialist. The reinvention of "family medicine" is in part a reaction to the perception that increasing specialization has been paralleled by an increasingly narrow clinical stance that renders the specialist insensitive to the needs and concerns of patients. The phrase "treating the whole person" strikes in many people chords of ambiguity, grandiosity, the overevaluation of existing knowledge, and unrealistic appraisal of the world we live in. But there can be no doubt that it is a phrase

---

[1]The reader who wishes a detailed description of what the clinical supervision of teachers entails should consult Goldhammer's (1969) *Clinical Supervision*. I know of no other book that even begins to deal with the nature, goals, and issues of clinical supervision with the comprehensiveness, creativity, and conceptual clarity displayed by Goldhammer. There is nothing in my experience to suggest that his book has had any influence on practice. What is so remarkable about Goldhammer's approach is how he obliterates the boundaries between the obligations to repair and to prevent.

that reflects a deep animosity to widespread insensitivity that people encounter with one or another kind of clinician; that is, the helper who approaches you with tunnel vision about what concerns you, what you fear, what you want to ask, what you define as help. If we look back with nostalgia on the physician of earlier times—for example, as Lewis Thomas (1983) does in regard to his physician father in *The Youngest Science*—it says a good deal about the roots of the resentment that people feel about the relative lack of caring and compassion. It is animosity captured well by Woody Allen's observation that "Not only is God dead but try getting a plumber on Sunday."

In medical schools, the researcher has more status than the faculty member who does not devote him- or herself primarily to research; and the medical student who is eager for a research experience is rated higher than the one who seeks more clinical experience. As we shall see later, in law schools, students who opt for a clinical experience are not judged as highly as those who seek opportunities for in-depth scholarship. It is no different in schools of education. The fact is that in all of these instances the quantity and quality of clinical training (broadly conceived and realistic in terms of what practitioners in these fields will encounter) are disconcertingly superficial. In our universities, justified as they are and should be on the basis of the conditions they create to contribute to knowledge through research and scholarship, the clinical or helping endeavor is a relatively new "add-on," one with which few people in the university feel comfortable. Time is a limited and precious resource, and when it must be allocated among research, scholarship, classroom teaching, and clinical supervision, it is supervision that is, so to speak, low person on the totem pole.

When Flexner recommended that the faculty of the medical school should be scientists-researchers, he did not intend that it should be at the expense of the most intense and rigorous clinical supervision. Flexner did not understand that, in what was then the early development of the modern university, his recommendation would present serious obstacles to the quality of clinical supervision. In the case of education, let us not forget that it was about the same time that the preparation of teachers (really the field of education) began to be taken into our colleges and universities. It was a very reluctant acceptance, as it still is today, because teaching was not considered a profession; that is, grounded in a body of theory, research, and knowledge that informed practice. Teaching was considered an art, not a science, an amalgam of talents and sensitivities that some people had and some did not, and there was little reason to believe that it was "teachable." That was a view that William James held, but, far from demeaning teachers, James had the highest respect for those who had that hard-to-define amalgam without which the classroom was a dull affair. I find it both ironic and instructive that, at about the same time that James and others expressed the view that this hard-to-define amalgam was the most important ingredient in teaching—albeit not a very teachable combination of temperament, interpersonal sensitivities, and devotion to children—Flexner was saying precisely the same thing about the role of "insight and sympathy" in the medical student. The irony inheres in the fact that, in justifying placing medicine and education in the university on the basis of ensuring that they would develop a scientific base for practice, their proponents had little or nothing to recommend about what they considered crucial interpersonal qualities. They knew, or thought they knew, how to teach the subject matter, morality, and applications of science. As for those other crucial qualities, they had to fall back on hope, the dynamics of the "calling," and the liberating of the mind through an education that enlarged one's cultural horizons.

In the case of education, there was one towering exception to the prevailing view: John Dewey. More than anyone of his time, and as much as anyone today, he knew that, in the preparation of teachers the major task was how to wed conceptual understanding of children and pedagogy with caring and compassion in practice. When you read about the school that Dewey started at the University of Chicago in 1896 (for example, Mayhew and Edwards, 1966), it is obvious that, for Dewey, the artistry of the teacher inhered in the ability to transform conceptual knowledge into actions appropriate to the needs of children, as individuals and in collectivities. I do not think Dewey ever used the adjective *clinical* in discussion of the nature, goals, and responsibilities of teachers, but it is hard to read Dewey and not conclude that he had a most broad and sophisticated conception of the clinical role in which teachers inevitably found themselves. He has been criticized for overemphasizing a child-centered approach, but that criticism totally ignores the revulsion Dewey experienced and expressed about teaching devoid of caring and compassion for the feelings and needs of children. Dewey was child centered in the sense that he advocated teaching children, not subject matter, in the same sense that one expects physicians to treat a person and not a symptom. And if today most teachers and physicians still do not grasp these distinctions, it says less about them than it does about the clinical aspects of their training.

If teaching in a clinical role with troubled children is an obvious fact of classroom life for which teachers are poorly prepared, there is another situation in which every teacher finds him- or herself and for which they are not prepared at all. Unlike the first type of situation, which is narrowly clinical in nature in that the goal is to help in regard to a here-and-now problem, the type of situation we shall now discuss has prevention as its goal. As I have emphasized, precisely because of the knowledge gained from efforts of repair, the clinician has the obligation to use that knowledge for purposes of prevention. This situation can be approached by posing this question: Why do most teachers find talking to parents difficult, unsatisfactory, anxiety arousing, a situation they would dearly love to avoid, and one that not infrequently becomes conflictful? You could put the question in this way: Why do so many parents approach a meeting with their child's teacher with trepidation, the sense of inequality, and concern about what to say and what not to say or reveal? I am not talking about parent-teacher contacts on "parents' night," a ritual or charade where both sides collude to avoid any meaningful discussion. Whatever the merits of such a ritual, and they are few, they do not include meaningful discussion. I do not say this only on the basis of personal experience, because, over a period of forty years of being related in some fashion to schools, I have rarely heard a teacher or parent talk about these rituals other than as devoid of significant interpersonal contact.

Let me relate an experience typical of many I have had on those occasions when I have been asked to meet over a period of weeks with a group of teachers about issues of concern to them. Many issues are brought up, and one of the quite predictable ones is their contacts with parents. This issue comes up with such regularity and feeling that on one of these early occasions I found myself telling the group: "I have come to the conclusion that if I were to ask you to choose between one of two recommendations, I know which one you would be tempted to choose. The first recommendation is that you receive a thousand-dollar salary increase. The second is that you will never again have to talk to another parent." Unfailingly, my statement engenders that kind of nervous, self-conscious laughter that indicates that I have touched the jugular. My statement reflected no special wisdom on my part but rather the fact that these teachers made perfectly plain that any child the teacher considers to be a problem in the classroom has parents who want to be, or should be, or must be involved in a remedial course of action. In short, the teacher seeks contact with the parent *after* he or she has concluded that there is a problem. But "after" usually means not soon after but rather long after, and one of the reasons for the delay is the reluctance of the teacher to deal with parents from whom they tend to expect the negative consequences of a partisan stance. From the standpoint of the teacher, most parents are, when the interests of their child are at stake, subjective, overemotional, and uncomprehending (not unlike the way many physicians view their patients). Intuitively, teachers know that their task is not one of merely imparting information but one of gaining and sharing information that will suggest actions that can gain the commitment of teacher and parents. But that intuition, vague and inchoate as many institutions are, is not nurtured by the stance of caring and compassion, the stance that makes comprehensible and predictable the congeries of attitudes and feelings that parents experience when they know that their child is in trouble in a setting fateful for his or her future. It is a stance that should give rise to surprise and dismay if parents are unemotional, undefensive, and unquestioningly accepting of the information imparted and of unilaterally formulated recommendations. It is more than a stance characterized by verbal expressions of sympathy, caring, and understanding; it is one where, on the level of action, the process of helping always is determined by, among other things, the effort to comprehend how the situation is being interpreted and reacted to by the other person.

What do teachers experience when as parents they seek a meeting with their child's teacher to discuss issues that trouble them about their child's classroom learning and behavior? Or when their child's teacher initiates such a meeting for similar reasons? Frankly, these are not questions that I initially asked of teachers who were parents. They were questions that teachers brought up as confirmation of the point that teachers received no preparation for how to talk to, be with, and help troubled parents. And, with few exceptions, teachers as parents frequently come away from meetings with their child's teacher frustrated, angry, and resentful of being "talked down to." In this connection, I should note that I have got similar reactions from physicians when they have been in the role of patient either in another physician's office or in a hospital.

I have been dwelling on the repair aspect of the teacher as clinician. How might we think about teacher-parent relationships from a preventive orientation? Let us start with the assumption that parents have information and feelings about their children that they are willing to provide and reveal in a nonjudgmental context. (Obviously, the situation in which a teacher and parents are meeting because someone already has identified a child as a problem is a loaded one.) Let us further assume that the knowledge and feelings that parents can and wish to provide are important to teachers in regard to how they will think about and respond to the child in their classroom; that is, that this knowledge and these feelings should influence the substance and depth of the teacher's caring and compassion for the child. The phrase "understanding a child" is sloganeering if it does not imply overt actions powered by caring and compassion. Indeed, when you say you want someone to understand your child, you mean you want that person to act in ways that, initially at least, reflect sympathetic *acceptance* of the world of your child according to your lights. You do not want that understanding to stop with labels and categories. I should hasten to add that neither of the two assumptions implies that what parents convey about themselves and their child is valid and complete. However, valid or not, in whole or in part, these assumptions imply that parental knowledge and feelings are indispensable to the teacher if his or her actions are to be informed by understanding, caring, and compassion. I do not wish to create the impression that parent-teacher contacts inevitably possess the characteristics of a cold war, but neither do I wish to suggest that these contacts, even under nonjudgmental conditions, are interpersonally simple affairs in which goodwill is the major lubricant that dissolves the potentials for discord.

When is there a nonjudgmental context in which teachers and parents can meaningfully establish a relationship that may prevent problems? I would suggest that such a time is *before* the school year begins; that is, when it is known who the child's teacher will be. It is then that teachers and parents can meet not around a problem but around what parents and teachers need to know about each other and the child. But how does one state the purpose of the meeting? For example, the teacher could say: "You know your child better than I do. You know your child in a way that I do not and never can. You know the kinds of things and situations that turn your child on or off. You know your child's weak and strong points. What you know and can tell me is crucial to me as your child's teacher. Similarly, what I observe and learn about your child in my classroom will be important to you, and I need to feel free, as I hope you will, to meet from time to time, not because there is a problem, but because we need each other in the best interests of your child."

The reader should not regard this statement as an excerpt from a manual on how to establish teacher-parent relationships that can prevent or identify school problems. I am no believer in the magic of words or the effectiveness of recommended step-by-step procedures that too frequently result in empty

rhetoric at the expense of any real understanding of overall purposes and the obstacles to their realization. The statement is a
basis for making several points. The first is that you cannot
make that kind of statement unless you truly believe that what
parents think and feel is important and useful and that, in fact,
parents know their children in ways that you cannot or do not.
The second point is that, in making the statement, you indicate
that you are prepared to stay in touch with the parents other
than at those times when you have a question about their child.
That is to say, you take the initiative to talk to parents at times
and in ways that make it easy for them to initiate discussions
with you. In short, the overarching purpose is to establish a give
and take that is the antithesis of an adversarial relationship, that
is based on mutual responsibility.

What are the obstacles to initiating and sustaining such a
relationship? There are many, but two require emphasis. The
first obstacle is one we have met before in our discussion of
medical clinicians: It would take far more time than teachers
now have. The calendar of the school year and the organization
of the school day leave no time for initiating and sustaining
such relationships. Just as physicians say they have insufficient
time to act caringly and compassionately with regard to the
needs and feelings of their patients, school personnel claim that
they, too, have insufficient time to act in accord with what I
have suggested. No teacher or physician has ever articulated this
obstacle to me as justification but rather as explanation. If we
had more time, they say, we could be more caring and compassionate. That explanation, unfortunately, is invalidated by the
second obstacle: The preparation of teachers, even more than
that of physicians, is utterly deficient in regard to teacher-parent
relationships. Assuming that more time would be available, why
should one expect that the quality of these relationships would
thereby improve?

In reality, there is a third obstacle, which is the most dis-
heartening: The issues I have raised are not seen as problems in
the preparation of educators. In all of the many reports that
have come out in the past few years bemoaning the state of
public education and making recommendations, most of which

are in the category of reinventing the wheel, there has been absolutely nothing that even by implication recognizes the significance for training of the fact that teachers are clinicians whose role, perhaps uniquely, exposes the conceptual nonsense in separating repair and prevention. The assumption seems to be that, as in the case of physicians, those who seek a career in education have, among other things, the qualities of being caring and compassionate people. And, presumably, those who lack these qualities will be screened out through the selection process. The realities make a mockery of these assumptions. There can be no doubt that, as a group, educators, like any other group, vary enormously in their capacity to be caring and compassionate people. But caring and compassion are not things or essences in, on, or about individuals. They are concepts that refer to features of relationships between people in certain kinds of situations. When we say a person is caring and compassionate, we do not (or should not) mean that those qualities are manifest in all relationships that person experiences from the time of rising in the morning until falling asleep at night.

Caring and compassion are not programmed in genes. They are features whose situational specificity has been learned. If we are far from understanding how they are learned in regard to this but not that kind of situation, we are more secure about when they are present or absent in a particular relationship. The extent to which these features are influenceable or teachable is an open question. To assume that they are neither is, at this stage of our knowledge, to indulge ignorance or prejudice. And to make this assumption in regard to teachers is an egregious, insulting example of blaming the victim. Nothing has contributed more to the lowly status of teachers than the imagery of the teacher as an imparter of knowledge and an engineer of skill training. It is imagery totally at variance with what teachers experience and confront. If it is imagery they bring with them when they seek to become a teacher, the formal training they receive does next to nothing to disabuse them of that unrealistic imagery. The disillusionment begins when they take up the independent role of teacher.

The gulf between repair and prevention—the wastefulness

that is a consequence of that gulf—is nowhere more clearly in the picture than when we look at lawyers who are clinicians: the thousands who on any one day are dealing with the legal and psychological sequelae of divorce. If we do not ordinarily think of lawyers as clinicians, and if they do not think of themselves as clinicians, the fact remains that these lawyers are in the role of clinician. By their very nature, the processes of separation and divorce bring to the fore a variety of problems for a variety of people: the parents, children, grandparents, friends, and extended families. We are far more aware of the problems, actual and potential, of parents and children than we are of those not centrally in the picture; that is, in the lawyer's office. If we know anything about separation and divorce, it is that there are two kinds of problems: those that are already apparent and those likely to arise in the foreseeable future.

In short, there are problems that require a here-and-now clinical approach, and there are problems that are preventable, in part or in whole. Both types of problems require of the lawyer knowledge, understanding, and the willingness to act in ways that dilute the adverse consequences of here-and-now problems and will prevent the development of further problems. But to deal with both types of problems assumes that the lawyer not only comprehends these problems but has the security and training compassionately to take on the obligations of the clinical and preventive roles. That assumption is, of course, an invalid one. There is literally nothing in the training of lawyers that prepares them for either role. "Why should it be otherwise," the legal educator will argue; "we educate and train lawyers, not mental health personnel. Our curriculum is so fantastically tight that there are a lot of aspects of the law that are only superficially covered." That is true, of course, but no legal educator with whom I have spoken has ever attempted to deny that the lawyer is potentially in the position to ameliorate present and prevent future problems. Similarly, in my conversations with scores of parents who have gone through the processes of separation and divorce, the bulk of them made it clear that their lawyers, however well intentioned and "nice," were of no help to them with the irradiating social-personal consequences of separation and divorce. We are obviously not talking about a minuscule number of adults and children, or actual and potential problems that are easy to face or overcome, or problems that in our society we can expect to decrease in frequency in the future. We are talking about a large number of adults and children experiencing a process that appears in most participants to leave lifelong scars. If we are sympathetic to what the legal educator said, we, as individuals and as a society, have to accept a situation where the possibilities for repair and prevention are as obvious as they are ignored. To accept such a situation is, to say the least, economically wasteful as well as the antithesis of being caring and compassionate in that we consign many people to misery, frustration, and the sense of unwanted aloneness.

If it is understandable that a professional field will not want to stray from its accustomed boundaries, it is no less understandable to suggest that, from the standpoint of the societal welfare, those boundaries will have to be enlarged so that a new responsibility or emphasis will have to take priority over an existing one. It is appropriate here to mention briefly one of the few studies of lawyers in relation to divorce. This study, by Doane and Cowen (1981), had as its main purpose "to learn about family lawyers' interpersonal help-giving behaviors and attitudes." How much time do they spend dealing with divorce clients' emotional problems? What kinds of psychological problems do such clients present? How do attorneys handle these problems? And how do they feel about this aspect of the family lawyer's role? Data were collected from questionnaires completed by sixty-two practicing family lawyers (approximately half of those to whom the questionnaire was sent). All but one of the lawyers were male. Their mean age was forty years, and they averaged thirteen years of practice. Each handled on average twenty divorce cases per year. For my purposes here, the following findings are relevant:

1. As one would expect, the problems clients brought to lawyers were obvious and serious. The most frequent problems were anger to spouse, depression, problems surrounding immediate contact with spouse, problems with children, and emotional outbursts or crying.

2. Roughly 40 percent of lawyers' total talking time centered around divorcing clients' moderate to serious personal problems. Although lawyers considered it very important to engage such problems and used a variety of strategies to do so, "they neither felt entirely comfortable nor effective in the help-giving role."

3. "The high correlation between frequency of occurrence of problems and lawyers' judgments about their difficulty in handling is of considerable interest. In two structurally analogous situations, teachers and nonprofessional child-aides judged the *in*frequent problems of young maladapting schoolchildren to be *more* difficult to handle than frequent ones. For lawyers working with divorce clients the reverse was clearly the case. That finding suggests that lawyers spend considerable time dealing with psychological problems which *they* judge to be difficult, and sometimes find to be 'over their heads.' Although they refer roughly 3 of every 20 divorce clients to mental health professionals, on the average only 1 follows-up."

4. "Some might argue that lawyers should not get involved in people's personal problems because they are not trained for such work. That view, however, flies in the face of the present data which establish clearly that—like it or not—they *are* so involved. Indeed, the special 'ecology' of the lawyer-client dyad often demands that that happen."

Doane and Cowen emphasize that, in regard to lawyers, "A vital missing link in the present picture is that we know little, if anything, about their *actual* effectiveness." In short, the data were obtained from responses to questionnaires, not from systematic observation. Are these lawyers caring and compassionate? Do their "response strategies" reflect a serious desire to understand and to take those actions of repair and prevention that such understanding suggests? If we were able to observe directly their behavior, is it more or less likely that we would be satisfied that the potentials for repair and prevention had been realized? If we cannot answer these questions about lawyers, neither can we answer them about physicians, teachers, and other clinicians. Until we are better able to answer these questions, we have no basis for believing that the clinical endeavor as we know it—as it is reflected in practice—is as productive as the practitioner asserts or as the society requires, faced as society always is by limited resources. To the extent that the clinical endeavor remains narrowly focused on the individual (and usually a part of him or her), it impoverishes that endeavor and widens rather than narrows the gulf between repair and prevention. The clinician should be a person for whom the preventive stance is not an "add-on" to his or her thinking and actions, not a luxury to be indulged only when time permits, and not inconsistent with the goal of reducing individual pain, misery, and illness.

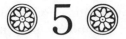

5

Examples
of Uncaring Behavior

It is a glimpse of the obvious to say that any pathological condition in an individual is social in the sense that it affects and is affected by the network of relationships in which the individual is embedded. By whatever criteria pathology is defined—and they may vary considerably in clarity, objectivity, validity, and even moral and cultural justification—the diagnosis immediately alters the thinking and actions of parts of the individual's social network.[1] Although that alteration is not necessarily negative in its consequences, it almost always is, and the question that immediately arises is: Who is the patient? That question is a justifiable one, even from a narrow clinical viewpoint, because, if an individual's conditions will have negative consequences for others, which in turn can have an unfavorable impact on that individual, the clinician is obligated to take this into account in both thinking and action. If all of this is obvious, and it has been obvious in the history of all clinical fields (indeed, since

---

[1] This is a point that was eloquently made by Richardson (1945) in *Patients Have Families* and by Engel (1977). Recently, in a special issue of the *Family Networker*, articles by Dym and Berman (1985), by Glenn (1985), and by Baird (1985) reiterate the point. Dym and Berman state: "In the initial excitement of the reevaluation of modern medicine, however, this most basic idea has gotten lost for a century or so. Now, there are so many forces at work in our society encouraging a return to a more integrative view of illness that such a shift seems inevitable." I am just as impressed with the forces that have been and continue to be obstacles to such a shift. Dym and Baird give no basis for their optimism.

the beginning of recorded human history), actions consistent
with the obvious either are absent or are token gestures. The
"who is the patient" question is no less justified from the standpoint of primary and secondary prevention, because, if you
know that an individual's condition will adversely affect and be
affected by the actions of others, how do you justify not seeking to prevent or to dilute negative consequences? Few things
are as effective in buttressing a narrow clinical and preventive
stance as the customary imagery of *the* individual with *the* clinician. It is imagery that is based on a fact that obscures the
truth. The fact is that the individual has a problem and requires
help; the truth is that problems beget problems, and solutions
beget problems; that is, as my colleague Dr. Murray Levine
felicitously put it: problem creation through problem solution.

Several explanations can be advanced for this view that is
so narrow in thinking and solution. The first implicates the narrowness of clinical training that rivets on the individual. The
second, a variant of the first, draws attention to the fact that
the knowledge and skills required to diagnose an individual's
condition are not the same as those required to deal with the
consequences of that condition for those in the person's social
network who will clearly be affected by (and who will in turn
affect) the condition. The third explanation points to the practical, inexorable effect of time as a limited resource; that is, the
clinician simply does not have the time to cope with these consequences with the same effectiveness as he or she does with the
patient as a single organism. This explanation, the most frequently expressed of the three, has always struck me as strangely revealing in that it attributes a degree of knowledge and skill
to the clinician at the same time that it is a justification for not
being able to apply that knowledge and skill. This explanation
becomes more suspect when one hears clinicians say that their
preparation was inadequate for dealing with the ripple effects of
the individual's condition and then go on to suggest that, indeed, their preparation was adequate, but limitations of time
preclude utilizing what they know and what they can do.[2]

---

[2] The words *ripple effect* conjure up imagery that is misleading in
that the ripples move in one direction: outward. The effects of the person

The three explanations, of course, deserve discussion, but I reserve that for a later chapter. What I seek to do here is to describe a condition that is frequent, that is always upsetting, whose transactional nature is clear, and whose goals of repair and prevention are obvious in their significance, but a condition that very frequently is handled in ways that no one would describe as caring and compassionate. It is also a condition that at some time or another, and sometimes at the same time, involves physicians and teachers. The condition I refer to is mental retardation, one that is sometimes apparent at birth but more often than not is discerned within the first few years of life. In our society, at least, few things are as upsetting to one's stance toward the future, or as bewildering to one's sense of parental competence, or as influential in the pressures exerted on parental relationship and life-style, as the news that one's infant or young child is mentally retarded. Many readers of this chapter are not parents, many readers are parents, but I am confident in asserting that every reader will feel sorry for parents who have just been given the diagnosis. The word *sorry* is related to the word *sorrow,* for which my dictionary says: "deep distress and regret; a cause for grief and sorrow; a display of grief and sadness." Intuitively, we have an exquisite sense of what these parents will think and feel. We do not have to be taught to feel sorry for people who have just learned that their child is mentally retarded. It is not an instance of joyous tidings. Granted that parents vary considerably in their response to the diagnosis in terms of short- and long-term consequences, I have never seen or heard of an instance that was not experi-

---

with a pathological condition are always transactional in that he or she affects and is in turn affected by others. Just as the relation between the clinical and individual is transactional, so is the relation between the individual and others in the family and social network. If I emphasize the transactional nature of human relationships, it is less for purposes of precision or verisimilitude and more because of what it implies for actions geared to helping. I have always found it fascinating that the transactional nature of relationships was crucial to the thinking of two people who profoundly influenced our world and who were markedly different from each other: John Dewey and Sigmund Freud. Whereas Freud stressed the transactional (transference-countertransference) in the analyst-patient dyad, it was conceptualized and applied far more broadly by Dewey.

enced by the parents, initially and for some time, catastrophically.

These introductory comments may have aroused puzzlement in the reader, taking the form of this question: How can you say that people intuitively feel sorry for these parents and also say that it is a situation that physicians and teachers often handle in uncaring and uncompassionate ways? Let us return to this question after I have described some characteristic experiences of some parents of mentally retarded individuals. These parents have in common the fact that they enjoy professional status; for example, psychologist, physician, schoolteacher. What I shall now report is based on *Parents Speak Out,* by Turnbull and Turnbull (1979), who are themselves parents of a retarded individual.

One of the chapters is by Dr. Phillip Roos, a psychologist who, before becoming a parent of a retarded child, had written and lectured on parental reactions to such a situation. The first problem he discusses centers around the fact that the pediatrician, in contrast to Dr. Roos and his wife, did not feel that there was anything wrong with their child. And then,

> Clinging stubbornly to the conclusion that our daughter was "probably just fine," our pediatrician next referred us to a neurologist. Since this worthy was a consultant to the large state institution of which I was the superintendent, I felt confident that he would immediately recognize the obvious signs of severe retardation in our child. Imagine my consternation when, after failing to accomplish even a funduscopic (vision) examination on Val due to her extreme hyperactivity, the learned consultant cast a baleful eye on my wife and me and informed us that the child was quite normal. On the other hand, he continued, her parents were obviously neurotically anxious, and he would prescribe tranquilizers for us. I had suddenly been demoted from the role of a professional to that of "the parent as patient": the assumption by

some professionals that parents of a retarded child are emotionally maladjusted and are prime candidates for counseling, psychotherapy, or tranquilizers. My attempts to point out the many indications of development delays and neurological disturbances were categorically dismissed as manifestations of my "emotional problems." I was witnessing another captivating professional reaction—the "deaf ear syndrome": the attitude on the part of some professionals that parents are complete ignoramuses so that any conclusion they reach regarding their own child is categorically ignored. Later I found that suggestions I would make regarding my own child would be totally dismissed by some professionals, while these same suggestions made as a professional about other children would be cherished by my colleagues as professional pearls of wisdom. Parenthetically, when I wrote to the neurologist years later to inform him that Val's condition had been clearly diagnosed as severe mental retardation and that she had been institutionalized, he did not reply [pp. 14-15].

I did not present this excerpt to make the point that physicians make errors in diagnosis. They do, of course, and this happens all too frequently in regard to mental retardation. The purpose of this excerpt was to illustrate an even more frequent phenomenon: the physician's uncaring, uncompassionate attitude toward parents. For the sake of argument, let us assume that Dr. Roos and his wife were flagrantly "emotionally maladjusted" and in need of tranquilizers and psychotherapy. Does that in any way justify the neurologist's blunderbuss attack on the parents? Does it justify literally adding insult to injury? Does it justify confusing telling the truth with being helpful? What is at issue here is not a technical problem—how to communicate the diagnosis. What is at issue here is one's comprehension of the meanings that parents will attach to information that is inevitably upsetting and disorganizing. And by *compre-*

hension I mean that almost unreflective sense that one accepts, appreciates, and is prepared for the consequences of the fact that what parents need at the moment is caring and compassionate behavior. That does not mean that you avoid telling the truth as you see it; it does mean that you strive to express in words and action that what the parents are thinking and feeling is understandable to you, that, if you were in their place, you would feel as they do. To accept and appreciate what parents think and feel is not only to give them what they most need at that time; it is the beginning of a process the goal of which is to intertwine two worlds: that of the parents and that of the clinician. To put it negatively, the goal is to avoid the feeling in clinician and parents that they are strangers to each other.

In a chapter by a physician, Dr. Leah Ziskin, she says:

> The worst statement or the statement that evoked the worst emotional response in me was "Don't worry, dear, everything's going to be fine." It took every ounce of will power and every lesson on tact and diplomacy that I had ever learned to contain myself and not shout back at anyone who said this, that I had reason to worry and that things were not going to be fine [pp. 74-75].

You might be tempted to say that telling parents that everything will be all right reflects far more caring and compassion than what was said to Dr. Roos and his wife. That conclusion, however, is unwarranted if by caring and compassion you mean accepting, appreciating, and willing to deal with the substance and consequences of what parents think and feel. As Dr. Ziskin makes painfully clear, being told that everything will be all right further deepens the well of frustration: "You do not understand!" Telling parents that everything will be all right is at best an indulgence of cheerful superficiality and at worst a reflection of an inability or unwillingness to be caring and compassionate.

Another excerpt is from the chapter by Ann Turnbull, a trainer of teachers:

Living with problems associated with mental retardation has substantially broadened my perspective of issues which must be addressed by professionals in interacting with families. Most formal training programs are extremely limited in preparing professionals to interact meaningfully with parents of retarded children in helping them solve very practical, day-to-day problems. In my formal training at three different universities, I cannot recall considering issues such as guardianship, helping brothers and sisters of retarded children understand the nature and implications of their siblings' handicap, helping retarded children make friends in their neighborhood and community, and ways to handle situations in public when strangers stare at and mock a retarded person. . . .

As a teacher trainer, I have substantially reordered priorities in preparing students to work with mentally retarded persons and their families. One project which evolved from the reoriented priorities was carried out in the course, Psychology of Mental Retardation, which I taught to juniors. Rather than having students do the routine term papers or journal abstracts, I required them to develop a one-to-one citizen advocacy relationship with a retarded individual and to keep a diary of their experiences, questions, insight, and concerns. The advocacy relationship was to be like a friendship involving activities such as participating in community recreation opportunities, going shopping, riding public transportation, preparing meals together, listening to music, constructing art projects, providing respite care, or simply visiting with each other. The advocacy projects proved to be a powerful training tool. The students reported learning far more from experiential contacts than from traditional methods of instruction. The first-

hand opportunity of getting to know a retarded
person and his family as people rather than as students or clients enabled the special education
trainees to become aware of some of the complex-
ities of handicapping conditions that are rarely
considered in university courses.

What goes on in training programs in the
name of education is sometimes shocking. It has
become very prevalent in special education departments of colleges and universities to offer courses
on working with parents. I cringe at the thought of
some of the course syllabi I have reviewed. In
many of these courses, very limited attention is
directed toward helping parents solve the day-to-
day problems which almost invariably are encountered, yet weeks are devoted to the "psychological
insight approach to parental guilt." Many such
courses are a fraud and tend to insure further conflict and unsatisfactory relationships between parents and professionals. Extended practicum with
families of handicapped children and the provision
of respite care for families should be standard requirements for courses which purport to prepare
students for working with parents [pp. 137–138].

Finally, the excerpt that follows is from Burke's chapter:

When Becky was one year old, we moved to
Gainesville, Florida. Our pediatrician in Billings
had sent a letter of referral to Shands Hospital at
the University of Florida. Our first visit to this
large teaching hospital for Becky to be examined
by the pediatric cardiologist and another, later visit
to the same place for an examination by the pediatric neurologist are among my worst memories.

We arrived at the hospital at 8:00 a.m. and
spent the whole day there. I filled out pages and
pages of forms and questionnaires as I juggled my

wiggly daughter. We were sent from this lab to that with instructions to "go to the third floor, turn left at the desk, go down three doors, turn right, and hand these cards and this form to the girl at the desk there," etc.

About 10:30 a.m. we were furnished with all the lab tests and were told to return to the pediatric cardiology clinic. There we were placed in a small examining room and I was told to undress Becky again and wait for the doctor. At 12:30 I went out to the desk and asked the nurse if we could go and get some lunch. They assured me that the doctor would come soon. A little later, after Becky had drunk several bottles of water (I had brought only one bottle of juice for her) and wet all the diapers I had brought for her, I asked the nurse to hold Becky for me for a minute. I couldn't lay her on the table or the chair because she'd fall and the floor was too cold to put her there. The problem was that I had to go to the bathroom and I didn't think I could manage it with Becky in my arms. The nurse grudgingly agreed but insisted I must be back in one minute. This episode increased my already rising feelings of anxiety and helplessness in this cold, impersonal place.

About 1:30 the resident physician came in and listened to Becky's chest and asked me some questions. He mentioned that she had a heart murmur. My fear and nervousness increased. At 3:00 the cardiologist came in and examined my sleeping daughter. She called the resident and asked him to listen to Becky's heart again and said "Where's your murmur now?" I hoped she was the one who was right.

After the cardiologist finished examining Becky, she told me that she had a normal EKG and her heart was a little enlarged which she assumed was the result of her earlier problems. She said that whatever problems Becky had had at birth had apparently corrected themselves. She advised us to return in one year for another checkup.

Then I asked her about Becky's motor development. She was over a year old and still couldn't sit up or crawl. I pointed out how stiff her legs were and how she stood on tiptoe when I stood her up. I explained that I had asked our family doctor about this and that he had told me that many children walk on their tiptoes when they are first learning to walk. She said, "I don't deal with legs, only with hearts, but if you are concerned about this, why don't you make an appointment with pediatric neurology? They are the ones who would deal with this sort of thing." She assumed that we could return the following week for such an appointment. She went out to the desk and said to the receptionist, "Please make an appointment for Mrs. Burke with pediatric neurology for next week." The receptionist laughed and said that the earliest appointment available would be in about eight weeks, so we took the earliest possible appointment.

From the vantage point of several years later, I am utterly unable to believe that the cardiologist did not know, or at least suspect what the problem was. I guess she didn't see any point in telling me that it was indeed an indication of a serious problem. By saying what she did, she avoided all discussion. It was frustrating for me to have to wait for an answer to that fearsome question, what is wrong? I think now that it is so painful to be the bearer of such dreadful news (that a child may have a permanent handicapping condition) that physicians avoid any discussions of this sort whenever possible [pp. 86–87].

Fairness requires that I state that the book *Parents Speak Out* is not a catalogue of horrors in which parents do nothing but vent their spleen at clinicians seemingly devoid of the ability to be caring and compassionate. Needless to say, although clinicians do not come up smelling like roses, these highly educated and articulate parents distinguish for the reader the difference between caring and uncaring clinicians and settings. However much the accounts of these parents-contributors differ in detail and emphasis, each of them criticizes the frequency with which caring and compassion is absent from clinician behavior, and each emphasizes the inadequacies of the training of clinicians.

There is a problem in drawing conclusions from the book edited by the Turnbulls, and, rather than state the problem, I will illustrate it by analogy to another frequent medical situation: the individual with cancer. One of my graduate students was married to a locally well-known and highly respected cancer specialist. What was remarkable about this physician was the gulf he experienced between the interpersonal support he gave to patients and what he wanted to give but felt he did not know how to give. He did not blame external factors. It was *his* problem, and the solution somehow had to come from within him. He was also a specialist in the inadequacies of his medical training for dealing with the social-familial-psychological consequences of learning that one had a cancerous condition. The reader does not have to perform a great leap of faith to assume that Dr. Leonard Farber was a caring and compassionate person who was not satisfied with how well his actions reflected these motives. The three of us discussed the issues and decided that it would be fruitful if we could make direct observations of his transactions with his patients. We worked out a simple observational schedule, permission for his wife (my student) to be present at examinations was obtained from patients, and observations were made of all patients who had appointments during a particular week. The most striking finding had to do with the amount of time devoted to a patient. Those patients who, like parents-contributors in the Turnbull book, were highly educated people received twice as much time with Dr. Farber as did those with a high school education or less; furthermore, the former far more than the latter asked questions and received answers.

The reason I refer to this unpublished study is to suggest that the level and quality of caring and compassionate behavior among the clinicians with whom parents of retarded individuals interact may be *overstated* in the Turnbulls' book. The parents in the Turnbull book, as is clear from reading the book, were or became very assertive people in response to the insensitivities they encountered. Most parents of retarded individuals, especially as one goes down the social-class scale, retreat from these encounters further into their private worlds of discouragement and despair.

The Turnbull book is an instance of a genre of publications in which a family member expresses frustration and outrage deriving from experiences with diverse kinds of clinicians, mostly physicians, and the settings of which they are a part. There has been a veritable explosion of these publications in the post–World War II era.[3] Mental retardation, autism, alcoholism, psychosis, learning disabilities, cardiac conditions, terminal illnesses, geriatric conditions—in regard to these and other conditions, some family member has been impelled to resort to print to describe, among other things, the percolating consequences of clinical behavior seemingly devoid of caring and compassion. When, as I discussed in an earlier chapter, medical educators cyclically bemoan the dilution of caring and compassionate feeling and action in physicians, they are not making a mountain out of a molehill. But their critiques apply to more than the medical clinician. And, I hasten to add, and as the report of the medical educators so clearly states, the problem inheres in the socialization process whereby the student is shaped for the clinical role. To blame the individual clinician is akin to blaming the victim.

---

[3] It is certainly not fortuitous that the field of family therapy also exploded in size and variety in the post–World War II era. Almost all the ingredients for a theoretical rationale for family therapy existed long before this era, but then, as is still the case today, mental health clinicians were imprisoned in an individual psychology that impoverished their effectiveness as repairers and preventers. The forces contributing to the growth of the family therapy field were and still largely are outside those centers in our universities where diverse clinicians receive their training.

A note now about how an unreflective or uncritical belief in progress can distort your assessment of reality. In 1949, I
wrote a book entitled *Psychological Problems in Mental Deficiency* (Sarason, 1949). It enjoyed a rather favorable reception
and was used widely in courses for diverse types of clinicians.
One of the chapters went into some detail on how one should
relate to parents in regard to the nature and consequences of
the diagnosis of mental retardation, emphasizing how the clini-
cal-preventive approach must start with a sympathetic affective-
conceptual understanding of parental phenomenology. So, for
example, I point out that you have to expect that many parents
will not want to accept what you are telling them and that
they will want to go elsewhere. Not only is that predictable, but
it should be accepted by the clinician, who should give the parents the names of other clinicians or agencies competent to render another opinion. That is to say, far from trying to persuade
parents that their quest should stop in your office, you should
suggest what you would want a clinician to do for you in a comparable situation—that is, to encourage and make it easy for parents to get another opinion, to make it possible for them to return to you if that is what they should decide. That chapter
derived from the fact that I had been spending a great deal of
time working with parents, many of whom (not all) had been
made to feel ignorant, incompetent, self-deluding cure seekers.
In any event, I had reason to believe that many clinicians in
training had found that chapter instructive and helpful.

Although, after the publication of the book, I remained
very much related to the field of mental retardation, I was no
longer in direct clinical contact with parents. For reasons that
to this day I still cannot fathom, I assumed that the situation I
had been writing about was on its way to getting "better and
better," that is, that parents were being responded to with more
caring and compassion than in earlier decades. So when, with the
aid of John Doris of Cornell University, the book containing the
chapter on interacting with parents was thoroughly revised, I
deleted that chapter. As soon as that new edition came out, I
heard from colleagues around the country, most of whom spent
a good deal of time working directly with parents, criticizing me

for leaving that chapter out. No one likes to be told that he or she has wrongly interpreted the status of a problem in the field. I began again to talk with parents, look again at the more recent literature, and talk to knowledgeable colleagues. If you were the kind of person who saw the bottle as half full rather than half empty, you might have concluded that physicians were manifesting no less a degree of caring and compassion than in the previous decade. At the least, clinicians in diverse fields were writing more and more pointedly about their responsibilities and ways of relating to parents. But overall, and especially in regard to practicing clinicians, I had to conclude that the situation was slightly improved but certainly not to the extent that justified my deletion of that chapter. I could not disagree with Wolfensberger's and Kurtz's conclusion in 1969 that "the story of the handling of parents of the retarded by professionals is a very sad one. While many unfortunate episodes have been the result of ill-advised but well-meaning management, others have been due to callousness and outright malpractice." Wolfensberger was speaking on the basis of a good deal of experience.

What do parents of retarded children look for in casting professionals in the various roles of service providers to their children? That question, as Huang and Heifetz (1982) note, has hardly been studied, and they go on to say that "many important questions regarding the nature of the parent-professional relationship remain unanswered. For example, the very basic issue of the parents' conceptions of helpfulness and their perceived and experienced roles in a helping relationship have not been systematically examined." The parent study attempted to gain a better understanding of parents' conceptualizations of "helpfulness." Huang and Heifetz developed a methodology that allowed mothers to provide qualitative and quantitative data about their experiences with the "most helpful" and "least helpful" professionals. Physicians and educators were by far the most frequently mentioned professionals with whom the parents had had a relationship. For my present purposes, several of the findings are most relevant here. First, medical professionals made up 35.7 percent of the "most helpful" category and 71.4 percent of the "least helpful" category. Second, analysis of the rating scales indicated that, of the ten characteristics that showed the greatest difference between most helpful (MHP) and least helpful professionals (LHP), most involved a general quality of warmth, concern, and support. Third, in answer to questions contained in the interview schedule, MHPs were "typically recalled as being 'interested,' 'concerned,' 'understanding,' and 'sensitive,' while the LHPs were 'discouraging,' 'insensitive,' and 'cold' and 'businesslike.' " This study, as these investigators explicitly state, is significant less for what it describes and explains than for the basis it provides for the recommendation that parental conceptions of and experiences in the helping relationships should receive far more systematic study than they have received. In the post–World War II era, there has been an unprecedented increase in the numbers and types of clinicians, in monies expended for services and programs, and in level of support for research on the evaluation of myriad aspects of the clinical endeavor. In light of these increases, is it not surprising that we have so few hard data on the characteristics of least and most helpful clinicians, and that, in these days when it is so fashionable to wave the flags of accountability and cost-benefit analysis, we have even less information (or systematic thinking, for that matter) on the psychological and financial price we pay for professional behavior that neither repairs, dilutes, nor prevents personal misery?

Although this study is obviously relevant to caring and compassionate clinical behavior, it is important to note that Heifetz (for example, 1980), more than anyone else, sees these characteristics in relation to what their absence may mean for mammothly delimiting resources vital to the goals of repair and prevention. So, for example, Huang and Heifetz (1982) found that, in contrast to the least helpful professionals, the most helpful professional "valued and applied the mothers' ideas in a genuine *spirit of partnership*. . . . In this regard, it is important to consider the recently accumulating evidence of parents' ability to carry out a wide range of educational and therapeutic functions for their own children. This represents a potentially dramatic increase in the quality and quantity of developmental resources available to retarded children. Tapping this vast potential would seem to require professionals who are generally supportive of parents, who acknowledge parents' current knowledge and capacity, who have specialized training and experience to complement the parents' expertise in their own children, and who are prepared to help interested parents further develop their own potential as service providers. These qualities are precisely the ones that mothers in this study emphasized in distinguishing the 'most helpful' professionals from the 'least helpful.' "

The acid test for caring and compassionate actions is when, as a clinician, you must deal with an individual or a situation foreign to your experience and your values—that is, foreign to your "shoulds and oughts of living." Concretely, how should a clinician—and in this instance, one could substitute the great bulk of lay people—respond to parents who seek his or her help in legally adopting a severely mentally and physically impaired child? Up until a few years ago, clinicians (physicians, psychologists, social workers, educators, lawyers) would have responded in two ways. First, it was impossible either on legal grounds or as a matter of stated public policy to arrange for such an adoption. That would have been the "matter of fact" and, therefore, the easy answer. The second response would have been: "Why on earth would you want to adopt such a child?" Accompanying this overt response would be the covert one: there must be something seriously wrong with people who want to adopt such a child. Why would anyone want to take on the responsibility of rearing a severely handicapped child who very likely will always be dependent on others for care and even survival? The possibility that there are people willing to adopt such a child precisely because no one else has the compassion to regard such a child as a human being deserving of care and love, who are more concerned with giving of themselves to such a child than with what they will get—that possibility has been and still is inordinately difficult for clinicians to entertain outside a framework of psychological pathology. That difficulty does not derive only from the fact that clinicians cannot imagine themselves doing what these parents seek to do. Clinicians frequently are faced with the actions of others that they themselves would not undertake, but clinicians are expected to get into the world of others in order to appreciate how those actions are embedded in a context of perceptions, purposes, and experience. In the case of parents seeking to adopt a severely mentally and physically handicapped child, it has been virtually impossible for clinicians to engage in the process of appreciation, because it is one powered by a caring and compassionate stance that, in these instances, is effectively short-circuited by an antithetical stance that gives rise to pejorative judgments. Far from attempting to appreciate, they depreciate. Nothing in what I have said is intended to convey the impression that the task of the clinician is to appreciate what parents seek to do *and* then help them do it. (Sometimes yes, and sometimes no—which is why the task of the clinician is and should be bedeviled by the ambiguities and dilemmas attendant to actions affecting the lives of people.) What I am saying is that the initial and crucial task of the clinician is to engage in the process that starts with caring and culminates in compassionate understanding of another person's phenomenology.

The world does change, albeit very slowly in regard to the legal adoption of severely handicapped children. Within the past decade, and for reasons having very little to do with changing attitudes in clinicians, such adoptions are not only permitted but encouraged. A recent study by Stone (1982) of eighteen sets of parents who had adopted such children is inspiringly instructive in regard to caring and compassionate behavior. Needless to say, as a group, these parents encountered in others (for example, friends, extended family) attitudes critical of adoption. But what comes through most clearly from these interviews is that these parents had a sense of mission and transcendence. It is as if they had a "calling" to rear, protect, and love an individual who otherwise would be the victim of all the consequences of societal indifference or rejection. As a group, they very consciously were wedded to a religiously informed sense of compassion. As one parent said: "I know that God would not give me a child I was unable to handle. He would give me the strength to do a good job" (p. 69). There was no evidence in the interviews that these parents suffered from a martyr complex or had un-

fulfilled reservoirs of masochism or in any way acted impulsive-
ly and self-indulgently. They did encounter numerous problems,
and there were strains on family relationships. But in the course
of the interviews—which varied from two to five hours in duration—no parent expressed regret at the decision, and, as a group,
they rated the adoption as successful. These parents did not
view their handicapped child as an object of pity but as someone who needed and could in some ways respond to caring and
compassionate actions.

     I trust that the reader understands that I have not used
Stone's study to suggest that these parents were in general more
caring and compassionate people than most of the clinicians
with whom they have had contact. In regard to their handicapped child, they were; but we should not be surprised if we
learned that in other situations these characteristics were absent. These are not characteristics that people are able to express in words and actions in all situations for which they are
appropriate. Though we may hope for such generalized consis-
tency, we do not expect it. But we should and do expect it of
clinicians, because it literally is their stock-in-trade, without
which their roles lack moral sanction. We expect that they will
fall short of the mark, but not to the extent that calls the endeavor into question. And that is the case today. The type of
situation Stone studied is but one of many that have forced individuals and groups within and without the clinical professions
to blow the whistle on what appears to be an increasing inability of clinicians both to appear and to act caringly and compassionately. As I said in early pages and shall pursue in a later
chapter, the problem is not one explainable (except in part) in
terms of the characteristics of individuals, as if socialization into
the clinical professions, the economics of clinical practice, the
corporatization-bureaucratization of the clinical endeavor, and,
for all practical purposes, the conceptual and actual separation
between the goals of repair and prevention are not major parts
of the picture. This is not to excuse insensitive clinical behavior,
just as one does not excuse illegal behavior because of a person's
unfortunate, deplorable, and personally corrupting background.

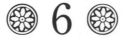

6

Psychiatry: The Caring and Compassionate Profession?

It is, at the least, ironic that, with the advent of war, a society begins to plan for the postwar care of casualties. Such planning reflects both moral and economic considerations. At the same time that the society seeks to provide rehabilitative care to those injured in the course of duty, it also assumes the responsibility financially to support, in whole or in part, veterans whose injuries will forever be with them. The staggering costs and moral dilemmas associated with the discharging of that responsibility became very clear during and after World War I, and, as soon as we became participants in World War II, serious planning for the care of veterans began. Although it was unclear whether the Allies would prevail, it was clear that, unlike World War I, this one would be long, would literally be worldwide, and would involve millions of people in the armed services. Indeed, it was obvious early on that the number of casualties would be of a magnitude far beyond what existing facilities and personnel could cope with. The federal government would have to underwrite not only a mammoth hospital-building program but a dramatic increase in the number of diverse types of clinicians as well. It is not much of an exaggeration to say that the federal government planned to underwrite an unprecedented rate of enlargement of American medicine and allied professions. Nowhere was the need greater than in those professions concerned with psychological disorders—psychiatry, psychiatric social work, clinical psychology and psychiatric nursing.

I have discussed elsewhere (Sarason, 1977, 1981) how social changes during World War II helped usher in the age of psychology or the age of mental health. Freud and psychoanalysis were legitimated in professional training programs in the university; in films, novels, and other types of national media, the public was exposed as never before to disorders to which the human mind was prey; Leonard Bernstein composed a concerto with the title *The Age of Anxiety*; and, in a few years after the war, the National Institute of Mental Health began a meteoric growth that, together with that of the Veterans Administration, was literally fantastic to someone who was in the mental health field before World War II. Psychology had arrived, the couch became more than a place for rest, it was chic to be in analysis, and, people were told, they should view personal problems in the same way you viewed any bodily ailment; that is, as something you go to somebody with for repair. The head of the department of psychiatry in a prestigious university got a lot of attention when he wrote a popular article in which he said that what we needed was psychotherapy for the masses at the rate of five dollars an hour! Inflated expectations were matched only by the economic inflation two decades later.

If, after World War II, psychiatry gained size, status, and institutional power, it was far from being a conflict-free environment. Indeed, it was a development that brought into the open psychiatry's long-standing problematic status in the medical school and medical education. As a specialty, psychiatry had long been low person on the medical school totem pole. That low status had numerous sources, but one of the most important for my present purposes was that psychiatry claimed, implicitly or explicitly (or was perceived as claiming), to have superior knowledge and skills in regard to understanding and changing human behavior; superior, that is, to the rest of the medical community. And, of course, that community did not take kindly to a message that suggested that their clinical skills—

their understanding of, relationship to, and management of their patients—not only were deficient in important ways but, to an undetermined extent, led to errors of omission and commission. No medical clinician has ever been known to state publicly that he or she is a bad psychologist. On the contrary, they pride themselves on their ability to "size up" a person; that is, to intuit his or her "psychology" and to take it into account in whatever course of action the person's condition requires. But psychiatry, derived as it is from some version of a general psychology, and relying as it does on a training that focuses on the understanding of human behavior, by its very nature clearly undercuts the claim of a nonpsychiatric clinician to psychological wisdom and skill. As a noted psychiatrist said to me: "No physician is born possessing psychological wisdom, and too many of them die without ever attaining it, in whole or in part." To which physicians would have replied: "Psychiatrists are poor physicians who mistakenly think they have cornered the market on how to understand and help sick people." Despite this mutual disdain, both camps agree about two things: understanding people requires experience and training, and without such understanding, caring and compassionate behavior is not likely to be manifested or effective. In light of the increasing concern of medical educators in recent decades about the lack of caring and compassion among physicians, the criticism by psychiatrists of their medical colleagues has received some confirmation.

The issue here is identical to that which exists in the university in the relationship between schools of education and the college of arts and sciences. Education has never enjoyed high status in the university, just as psychiatry has never enjoyed high status in the medical school. Indeed, schools of education have always been objects of criticism, often public and vitriolic, in the academic community. Although the reasons are many, one is truly basic: schools of education rest on the assumption that knowledge of subject matter does not guarantee effective teaching of that subject matter. The college of arts and sciences rests on the assumption that knowledge of subject matter guarantees, generally speaking, effective teaching of subject matters.

The two assumptions, of course, are irreconcilable. Similarly, a department of psychiatry rests on the assumption that sheer knowledge of theory and research—indeed, sheer experience—about human behavior in no way guarantees that it will be applied appropriately in the clinical interaction—in any clinical interaction, psychiatric or otherwise. More specifically, to the extent that clinical training in any medical specialty does not reflect a serious commitment (in formal courses and supervision) to psychological factors, it can seriously and adversely affect the clinician's ability to be appropriately caring and compassionate and, therefore, helpful. It should occasion no surprise if medicine generally views psychiatry as a haven of arrogance and professional imperialism.

But, in the post–World War II era, a new note entered psychiatric thinking, adding to the challenge that psychiatry represented to the medical community. Briefly, psychiatric thought began to reflect the impact of the social sciences in two major ways. First, the behavior of individuals was seen as influenced by and taking place in social-cultural-ethnic contexts. Put in another way, no longer could human behavior be understood in terms of a narrow individual psychology insensitive to the fact that our society was heterogeneous in major ways—socioeconomically, racially, religiously, culturally, educationally, and sexually. Sociological factors were more than just a basis on which one could break down populations into groups; these factors were assimilated by individuals, shaped their world views, and put a distinctive stamp on their behavior. To ignore these factors in an individual's psychological bloodstream set drastic limits to one's understanding of that individual's problems in living and to one's capacity to be helpful. And to the extent that this ignorance limited understanding or contributed to misunderstanding, it had obvious adverse consequences for the clinician's capacity to be appropriately caring and compassionate. But this was not a problem restricted to mental health clinicians. It was no less a problem for any medical clinician dealing with an ill individual: the nature and origins of the illness; the patient's understanding of the illness, ability or willingness to provide relevant information, and capacity to adhere to a treatment plan; and so on. If physicians had long paid lip service to the presence and importance of psychological factors in illness, the new psychiatry further undercut the medical clinician's claim to sophistication. In terms of understanding, prevention, and treatment, the physician-patient relationship took on a new conceptual and interpersonal complexity.

If the new "social psychiatry" represented a challenge to medicine generally, and not one endearing itself to that community, the fact is that the challenge of the social sciences to psychiatry was far from being greeted with enthusiasm, let alone general acceptance, within psychiatry. For one thing, as Grob (1983) has so well documented, up until World War II, psychiatry had striven valiantly to establish itself as a medical specialty in terms of both research and practice. The field very self-consciously became a "biological psychiatry." There were, of course, a few psychiatrists (for example, Harry Stack Sullivan, James Plant, Abram Kardiner) who, mightily influenced by some social scientists (for example, Edward Sapir, Harold Lasswell, John Dollard, and others in the "Chicago school"), swam against the mainstream; but, institutionally speaking, they had little influence. If the social upheavals produced by World War II brought into center stage the significances of cultural, racial, ethnic, social-class, and gender factors in the clinical and preventive endeavors—not only in psychiatry but in any clinical field— it should occasion no surprise if, again institutionally speaking, the dominant tradition in psychiatry could not digest the new orientation with anything resembling ease. Psychiatry became a divided camp. After all, the challenge to traditional psychiatry was identical to that of the clinical endeavor generally: to the extent that caring and compassionate behavior was based on an understanding of what I shall call for shorthand "social factors," it obviously had major implications for what clinicians had to know. But the challenge went further than that in the sense that it implicitly asserted that the degree to which the clinician could be helpful, and preventive efforts effective, was drastically lowered by ignoring these social factors. It was not that caring and compassion needed justification but that their content and behavioral consequences required a prior kind of understanding that, by its absence, had limited psychiatric effectiveness and, some argued, had had harmful consequences.

The conflict within psychiatry came into clear focus, as did a lot of other things, in the turbulent sixties. The inequitable distribution of health services (most blatant in psychiatry), racial conflict, the civil rights and women's liberation movements, the so-called sexual revolution, and the many other challenges to conventional wisdom and institutional authority converged, directly and indirectly, in the community mental health movement, manifested concretely (literally) in the development of community mental health centers. Funded as those centers were by federal and state grants, largely to departments of psychiatry, the power relationships between the biologically and socially oriented groups in those departments began to change. It was a struggle about power in that what was at issue was who would determine the education of the psychiatrist, the kind of research that would be encouraged, the populations to be served, and, always in the picture, the relation of psychiatry to the medical community. Whereas psychiatry had always oriented itself to gaining status in the medical school, the new breed of psychiatrist looked in two directions: the medical school and social science communities.

It is beyond my present purposes to go into detail about what happened in the sixties in regard to the community mental health movement. The institutional histories have yet to be written, although Levine's (1981) recent book may be a harbinger of what we may expect. I have discussed these matters in greater, although by no means exhaustive, detail in my book *The Psychological Sense of Community: Prospects for a Community Psychology* (Sarason, 1974). Suffice it to say that, if psychiatry's moving out into the social world was not a total disaster, it exposed in tragic and poignant ways how ill prepared, conceptually and clinically, psychiatrists were for dealing in new ways with new populations in a new setting. It might be more correct to say that what became obvious was how much a prisoner of tradition, biological and otherwise, the psychiatrist was and would increasingly become. Within the past decade, psychiatry again has become biological with a vengeance, and that is in no small part a reaction to the failures of the previous decades. Far from critically examining the sources of that failure, why its clinical efforts with heretofore unserved populations were generally ineffective, and why these efforts so frequently met with resentment and rejection, psychiatry reverted to a narrow biological tradition. Social factors, issues surrounding caring and compassion in the clinical interaction with diverse groups of people, the potentials of the clinical situation for prevention and repair—these have receded to an unlit back burner. Indeed, I have heard members of psychiatry departments seriously say that the entire psychotherapeutic endeavor should be given over to others (for example, clinical psychologists, social workers) and that psychiatry should concentrate on the study of the biological basis of human behavior.

Let us backtrack in order to gain perspective on psychiatry's efforts to change itself and to become more pervasively integrated in medical education generally. Illuminating in this regard is *Psychiatry and Medical Education* (American Psychiatric Association, 1952), a report of the 1951 conference on psychiatric education organized and conducted by the American Psychiatric Association and the Association of Medical Colleges. Although psychiatry had the most representatives, the social sciences and other medical specialties were also represented at the conference. There is nothing in the report to suggest that its major assertions and recommendations lacked the approval of all the participants. The report is very clearly written, it studiously avoids partisan narrowness, and, for the most part, it does not oversimplify issues, although its recommendations tend to be on a level of generality with which it would be hard for anyone to disagree. Perhaps the greatest significance of the conference was the recognition and acceptance it gave to the view that the physician had an obligation to understand and meet the psychological as well as the physical aspects of patients. It would be more correct to say that the conference reflected the fact that this view did not adequately or appropriately inform medical education. As in the case of the Flexner report, this conference was a response to a changing scene in psychiatric theory and practice and to changes in the larger soci-

ety: "industrialization, urbanization, suburbanization, changes
in value systems, secularization, migration, and changes in traditional institutions, notably the family. It is assumed that these
rapid changes may contribute to intensification of emotional
tension, anxiety, and conflict, to which many persons respond
with impaired health" (p. 124). Put most succinctly, the conference is inexplicable unless it is seen in the context of what
happened to psychiatry and the society during and in the immediate aftermath of World War II. Just as the Flexner report
of 1910 gave recognition to myriad scientific advances and their
implications for medical education, so did the 1951 conference
mirror the recognition of sea-swell changes in society as well as
in psychological (especially psychoanalytical) theory, heretofore minimally represented in academic psychiatry, let alone in
medicine generally. And just as the Flexner report was directly
and indirectly supported by major foundations eager to improve
medical education, so did the 1951 report have the financial
support of the federal government, increasingly responsible for
enlarging, improving, and funding medical education.

There are a number of assertions and recommendations in
the report that are relevant to the purposes of this book. I shall
restrict myself to a few of them. The first has to do with admission policies:

> The primary factor now governing admis-
> sion policies, it was generally agreed, is scholastic
> grades. Admission on the basis of grades means, in
> effect, on the basis of grades in the physical and
> natural sciences, and of interest and proficiency in
> things rather than people. Because high school and
> college counselors are impressed by the weight
> which medical schools give to preparation in the
> physical and natural sciences, they advise prospec-
> tive medical students—who tend to make a relative-
> ly early vocational choice—to take as many courses
> as possible in these disciplines. In addition, college
> requirements for a "major" or a field of concentra-
> tion often compel a pre-medical student to take

considerably more of one particular science than is required for admission to medical school, and this limits the courses he might otherwise take. As a result, applicants as a group are better grounded in the physical and natural sciences than in the social sciences and liberal arts. In other words, current admission policies seem to select students who will do well in the basic scientific aspects of medicine without sufficient regard for the more personal and social aspects [pp. 14–15].

The report goes on to say that grades should continue to be used, since "we do not know as yet what special qualities make a good medical student or a proficient physician, and thus do not have other criteria" (p. 15). Personal interviews, the report says, have no empirical value for purposes of prediction, because "every applicant knows enough to put his best foot forward during the interview and to cover up his liabilities." It would be desirable, the report continues, "to have a psychiatrist on the admission committee, or at least to have a psychiatrist take an active part in the work of the committee" (p. 15). And in regard to the college years, the report states:

Present medical education is too specialized, with undue weight on the natural and physical sciences. The balance between these disciplines and the social sciences needs to be improved. Courses in the latter field and in the humanities are desirable, not to give the student an appearance of culture but for their general educational value and to increase his understanding of people. Anthropology, sociology, psychology, English, history, and art were mentioned as among the studies that may lead the student to a greater understanding of people and hence be pertinent in his medical training. However, it was not urged by the Conference that any specific courses in this group be made formal requirements, because the value of any course de-

pends to so great an extent on the caliber of the
individual teacher.

The function of a liberal arts course, or any
college level course, is to produce educated men
rather than pre-professional technicians [pp. 17–
18].

It is a virtue of the report that it states in the most explicit way that future physicians, in contrast to those in the present
and past, have to be as understanding of persons as they are of
"things." One does not have to be adept at reading between the
lines to see that this assertion is prodromal of recent reports
about the lack of caring and compassion among physicians. It is
another virtue of the report that it identifies the blatant inadequacies of customary processes of selection and self-selection.
That virtue turns out to be empty in two respects: after indicting grades as a criterion, it reinforces their use, and after right-
fully undercutting the value of the interview, it goes along with
it if a psychiatrist can be part of the process, as if there were an
empirical base establishing that psychiatrists would enhance the
predictive value of the interview because of their presumed superior sophistication in sizing up people in a single interview.
Here again, one sees the not so implicit challenge that psychiatry represents to other medical specialties. Indeed, the recommendation that psychiatrists should participate in the interviews indicates that psychiatry was far from the apex of power
and decision making in medical schools. In saying this, I do not
think I am indulging in overinterpretation, and it certainly
squares with my own experiences in those years. Let it be
noted that, in the decades following the report, psychiatry's
status in medical schools took an upward course (for example,
psychiatrists are almost always part of the admission process),
and, as I described in an earlier chapter, the defects of the usual
selection and self-selection processes are more glaring and the
articulated concerns of medical educators more poignant. In regard to admission policy, the report states the problem, then
avoids it, and ends by essentially accepting the status quo. Quite
a contrast to Abraham Flexner's 1910 report, which someone

once characterized as "fighting words elegantly expressed." It should be noted that the last sentence in the preceding quotation is identical to the recommendation about the "educated man" made by Flexner in 1910.

It is, in my opinion, a justifiable act of faith to believe that liberal arts courses have "general educational value and increase understanding of people."[1] But that faith should not lead one to overestimate the depth and extent of understanding derived from what is predominantly book knowledge. Like Flexner, the report pins its hopes for the selection of caring and compassionate medical students—those, in Flexner's terms, with the requisite "insight and sympathy"—on the "educated man" appropriately influenced by a liberal arts curriculum. Selection and self-selection by this criterion were, if not decisive, very important.

The report never deals directly with why "present medical education is too specialized, with undue weight on the natural and physical sciences." How did this come about? What did this signify about the direction American medicine had embarked on? About American society? Was there any basis for believing that the recommendation about premedical education was sufficiently radical or innovative or even critical to prevent a bad situation from getting worse? If these questions are not addressed, it is because neither in psychiatry nor in medicine generally was there any tradition to view these enterprises in a self-consciously social-historical way. Not only could the past

---

[1] One sentence on page 14 of the report states that "Any restrictive admission policy in regard to geography, sex, race, religion, etc., has a deleterious effect on the caliber of the student body." What is implied but not said is that American medicine had long been characterized by a restrictive admission policy, against which Flexner had taken a firm stand. I note this obvious fact because this policy, far from contributing to the medical student's understanding of people, had the effect of narrowing that understanding and, therefore, adversely affecting his or her capacity to be caring and compassionate in regard to those of diverse cultural backgrounds. And that was no less true, of course, in regard to women, as became clear in the decade when the women's liberation movement began to pick up steam and took dead aim on, among other things, male-dominated medical attitudes and practices.

not be confronted, but the outlines of a future could not be drawn. The major goal of the report was elsewhere: to establish and solidify exposure to psychiatry in the medical school curriculum. *That* would be the major vehicle whereby the medical student would learn about the interrelationship among understanding, caring, and compassion. It proved to be too frail a reed, if only because the processes of selection and self-selection became even more narrow, and the ambience of medical training became increasingly characterized by training in technical skills, the accumulation of facts, the emphasis on laboratory research, and the "necessity" for narrow specialization. Something was happening on the way to the forum, but no one was taking notes.

As one might expect from a report on psychiatry in medical education, emphasis is placed on "the importance of personal relationships for success in becoming a doctor" (p. 12). That emphasis is buttressed in the following ways:

> It is evident from several studies of the characteristics of medical students, made particularly during the first year, that they are subject to a great deal of anxiety. If they can find faculty members or physicians in the student health service who seem to be sufficiently sympathetic, many will seek advice about their anxieties and emotional disturbances. If they do not find friendly acceptance somewhere in the medical school organization, there may be an intensification of their difficulties, possibly to the point of academic failure, or worse, of impairment of health.
>
> A few studies are available indicating the frequency of temporary or long-term emotional problems encountered among medical students. According to Fry and Rostow, relatively few medical students at Yale seek psychiatric help. Those who do so present mainly problems of indecision about their choice of a career or about curriculum requirements. Fry finds medical students as a group

rather hostile to psychiatric help. Studies at Cornell, Illinois, and Chicago reveal that about 25 percent of all medical students are in need of help for various emotional problems or psychiatric disabilities. In a study of a senior medical school class by Edward A. Strecker and colleagues, 46.5 percent were found to have neurotic handicaps of major character, constituting serious problems in mental hygiene.

A study concerning the problems of medical students at Illinois, conducted by Earley and Brosin, disclosed that about one-fifth of the students are psychiatrically ill to varying degrees of seriousness and another one-fourth have personal problems, but the amount of interference with their work is relatively minimal. Of the one-fifth that the authors would classify as having [a] severe degree of mental illness, some psychosis and some borderline psychosis is present. However, a large number of these are so-called character disorders, often unrecognized or only casually recognized by the individual.

A variety of factors operate as immediate stressful situations for the medical student in bringing out acute reactions or in exacerbating long-term reactions. Briefly enumerated they are: limited recreational and social outlets, fear of failure, highly competitive environment, conflicts over his dependent role, serious long-term sexual conflicts, and a sense of inadequacy in dealing with problems of patients.

Medical students, it is generally agreed, are exposed to a greater extent than most other students to situations likely to reveal personal inadequacy, immaturity, and anxiety. It was not, however, demonstrated that they constitute an atypical group. Indeed, some members of the Conference held that medical students are a typical cross sec-

tion of the American public in reflecting the
stresses and anxieties inherent in culture [pp. 12–
13].

Medical students may or may not be a typical cross section of the American public in regard to coping with personal
difficulties. As the preceding excerpt indicates, if they are typical, there is a problem, and if they are not typical, there is more
of a problem. If my experience—supported by many articles and
news reports in the national media—is any guide, in the decades
following the report, the level of competitiveness, ambitious-
ness, status seeking, material expectations, and anxiety among
premedical candidates as well as among medical students dramatically escalated. In short, it is my opinion that medical students are not a typical cross section of the American public in
regard to factors relevant to understanding people and using
that understanding in caring and compassionate ways. That
opinion, I should hasten to add, says as much (if not more)
about the culture of premedical and medical schools in American society as it does about students as individuals. Indeed, it is
conceptual nonsense to characterize these students as typical or
atypical independent of the educational cultures into which
they are socialized, a point well recognized in recent reports to
which I referred in an earlier chapter. It is a point made briefly
and mutedly in the 1952 report.

As one might expect, the report recommends that "Instruction in psychiatry in the first and second years of medical
training is desirable for the development of a mature professional perspective and a social approach to medical problems"
(p. 22). That recommendation is preceded by the following
statement:

Desirable changes in the first two years are
not a question of additions to or subtractions from
the curriculum, but rather a shift of focus. There is
need for less emphasis on information and the accumulation of a mass of factual data, and more on
how knowledge is discovered and put to use. At

present, the first two years tend to foster the idea
in the student that he is expected to be wholly a
scientist, whereas one of the important final objectives of medical training as a whole is the development of his skills in dealing with people.

If the development of skills in understanding and dealing with
people is such an "important final objective," why is the recommendation described as "desirable" and not mandatory? The
obvious answer is that the control and direction of the medical
school curriculum were and are in other departments far more
institutionally powerful and entrenched than psychiatry. And
among those departments, as anyone even slightly familiar with
medical schools will attest, there were and are competitive controversy and conflict about gaining, increasing, and protecting a
department's part of an already crowded medical school curriculum. If, therefore, the recommended changes were put forth as
"desirable," it was an instance of making a virtue of necessity.
If the report was realistic in this regard, it was unrealistic in its
assessment both of the willingness of the medical school to
adapt to other than tokenism and of the increasing momentum
in medical schools to emphasize a narrowly scientific-technological basis for medical research and practice. To the question of
what kind of person a physician should be, the report gave one
kind of an answer, and the traditions and customs of the medical school, so clearly formulated by Flexner, gave a different
kind of answer. Its deficiencies aside, the report is historically
important in several respects: pinpointing the problematic status of the selection and self-selection processes, the narrowness
of the medical school curriculum in regard to understanding
psychological and social factors in living generally and illness in
particular, the adverse effects (for example, in terms of personal
adaptation and values) that the medical school culture can have
on students, and the emphasis given to the assertion that the
recommendations made are applicable to all physicians-to-be
regardless of the medical specialty they choose.

The report says little about how the introduction of psychiatry into the medical school curriculum would be accom-

plished. It says nothing about why the usual pedagogical methods (lectures, demonstrations, case conferences) should be expected to accomplish even the modest goals stated in the report. I shall have more to say about this later. Let us turn now to *The Psychiatrist: His Training and Development* (American Psychiatric Association, 1953), a report of a conference held one year after the one I have just discussed.

Today that report has somewhat of an antique flavor, because it was written at a time when psychoanalysis was becoming a dominant focus in academic psychiatry in terms of theory, research, practice, and training. Within the next three decades, that focus became far less dominant, replaced by a return to a much more traditional biological psychiatry. Disenchantment with the promise envisioned by the proponents of psychoanalysis had many sources, which, although fascinating and instructive, are not directly relevant to my purposes. But that disenchantment, justified in part, at least, has had the effect of removing from center stage the most significant challenge that psychoanalysis presented to psychiatric training and practice. Put most briefly, that challenge was that to understand another person in ways that engender compassion for what that person experiences and how that person becomes what he or she is requires a degree of self-understanding not ordinarily attained in the course of living through customary courses, readings, and lectures. Freud, let us not forget, was crystal clear that what he was describing and conceptualizing was no less true for the treater than for the treated. Indeed, the 1953 report contains the following:

> Because psychiatry is fundamentally involved with processes of growth and failure in maturation, not only in patients but in ourselves, good teaching requires that the residents be helped to see in what way residues of their own infantile attitudes may block their work. The techniques of supervision, designed to help the residents to a better understanding of their own problems with patients, tend to foster the general attitude that

teachers are all adults, and "pupils" are all children who need guidance and help in maturing.

Another factor in this tendency to spoon-feed, to treat the resident as an immature pupil, is that the relative inadequacy of psychiatric training in undergraduate medical schools brings people into residency in various stages of ignorance and inadequate preparation. In an effort to rectify these deficiencies, there has been an acceptance of more elementary concepts of teaching that are somewhat inappropriate in a residency program [pp. 57-58].

If requiring psychiatrists to be psychoanalyzed was not practical and not always desirable, as the report recognized, and if, then or now, there is no compelling evidence that a personal analysis accomplished its major goals, the truly basic challenge that psychoanalysis represented (and represents) has been ignored as psychiatry has again become enamored with a biological, reductionist view of human behavior. The pendulum has swung from one extreme to another, from one type of narrowness to another. So, for example, the report recognizes that, self-understanding aside, the psychiatrist deals with people from backgrounds and perspectives clearly different from his or her own, differences that can be major obstacles to understanding, compassion, and appropriate forms of help. These are not issues and obstacles that are anything like central to the purposes of an analysis, although in practice they are very important, practically and theoretically. If the report recognized this, its emphasis on psychoanalytical theory all but overwhelmed that recognition. In regard to those issues, the report does recommend courses, seminars, and lectures on the social science aspects of psychiatric theory and practice. Although it would be unfair to describe this as tokenism, it had all of the consequences of it. Needless to say, in light of the pendulum swing, it is fair to describe the present situation as one of tokenism. The current prepotent tendency in psychiatry (and in medicine generally) to prescribe pills to alleviate personal distress and misery short-circuits the need to understand others or, for that matter, oneself. I am not asserting as a principle or a value that the use of drugs in matters of personal misery is unjustified. I am asserting that when they are used, as they too frequently are, as a means of first and not last resort, as a sustained form of "treatment," we should at least recognize that, as a field of clinical practice, psychiatry is running the risk, strange though it may sound, of losing the reason for its existence: contributing to knowledge about how understanding others, self, and major social-cultural contexts and differences shapes the substance and style of behavior and, therefore, should inform the clinical endeavor. I am not indicting an entire field. There are psychiatrists, not minuscule in number, who not only would agree with my criticism but would view it as a bit too moderate.

I have been in the field for over forty years, starting at a time when shock treatment was but one example of a dominant biological approach. I witnessed and participated in the internal struggles that were a consequence of the political legitimation of psychoanalysis in departments of psychiatry. There was never any doubt that what was at issue was less how to help people with personal problems and more the role of the psychiatrist's self-understanding in the helping process. No one, of course, was against self-understanding. The issue was the extent and depth of that understanding in regard to the diversity of types of people the psychiatrist encountered. From the standpoint of the 1953 report, that question was essentially answered by its emphasis on extent and depth. If there was any ambiguity on this score, let us listen to what the report says about the significance of self-understanding in the medical specialist who is not a psychiatrist:

> Whatever the specific content of the training and whatever the methods employed, there is an underlying expectation which may not always be realized, that the physician will be aided to develop an interest in and an understanding of people and their problems of adaptation, and respect for their potentialities for more constructive adjustment. He must be able to retain his own equanimity even in

the face of the patient's hostility and he must also
be willing to examine his own behavior and attitudes to discover elements that may have evoked
hostility. He must be patient, for it is often necessary to be content with little progress and to accept limited objectives while the patient is slowly
working through misinterpretations and poor decisions to a better adjustment. He must avoid expressing contempt, ridicule, or disapproval, directly or indirectly by word or gesture. He must keep
in mind that the patient may be guided, but that
he cannot be pressed into courses that are contrary
to his own attitudes. Above all, the physician must
assiduously avoid unconsciously using his patient
to work out his own problems and conflicts, or
dominating him to enhance his own feeling of security [p. 55].

If these were "underlying expectations" of the nonpsychiatric
physician, the expectations for psychiatrists were obviously
greater. The issue is, unfortunately, no longer a central one in
psychiatry. But, as I discussed in earlier chapters, it has been
raised again in regard to the dilution of caring and compassion
among physicians generally. And it is being raised not by psychiatrists but by lay people and some in other medical specialties. In the pendulum swing back to a reductionist, biological
orientation—becoming "real" doctors—one cannot unreflectively
exempt psychiatry from the current criticism. I do assume that,
as a group, psychiatrists are more caring and compassionate
than other medical groups, but that difference has become far
less than one expects from a comparison involving a group
whose raison d'etre is understanding the complex springs and
contexts of human behavior. I have been witness to too many
instances where dispensing drugs (sometimes in assembly-line
fashion) has become a substitute for the pursuit of understanding. It is one thing to make a virtue of necessity. It is quite another thing to forget why you are in business.

By what criteria should people be selected for training in

psychiatry? The report provides a clear answer: the usual methods (such as appropriate motivation, high standing in medical school, performance in psychological tests, screening interviews) do not distinguish between those who become good and those who become bad psychiatrists. Selection is discussed in three pages; alternatives to the usual methods are not presented. In the first sentence of the section, the report asks: "Once the candidate has been accepted for training, how does the milieu in which he finds himself affect him as a person, and what personal problems are inherent in the nature of the residency environment?" (p. 70). In light of that question, it is noteworthy that the report does ask a related question: Once a person has been admitted to medical school, how does the milieu affect him or her as a person, and what personal problems are inherent in the nature of the medical school environment? In the 1952 and 1953 reports, there are sentences, paragraphs, and sections that are implicitly and explicitly critical of the nature and consequences of medical school culture on the student's understanding of self and others and, therefore, on the quality of their relationship to patients. Put in another way, there is a wealth of observation that suggests that four years of socialization in the medical school culture are interfering with, not facilitating, the goals of psychiatric training outlined in the report. The adverse effects of that socialization have hardly been explored, despite their obvious implications for psychiatric training. Bearing in mind the fact that the major goal of socialization is to ensure continuity between generations, one cannot be optimistic that psychiatric training can dilute to a significant degree the adverse personal and professional-attitudinal consequences of the medical school experience. And the degree to which that dilution is possible is limited by another fact: psychiatry's striving to be an important part of the medical school culture, a striving that is best described by the psychoanalytical mechanism of identification with the aggressor. In the case of individuals and collectivities, striving for upward mobility is incompatible with radical thinking. The Faustian legend has a firm basis in human history.

Flexner's report was radical in the literal sense in that it sought to change the roots, so to speak, nourishing medical education. It sought to affect the selection process by requiring an extended college education. It aimed to change the characteristics of the medical faculty as well as the relationship between students and faculty. And, of course, it recommended sweeping changes both in the depth and breadth of the curriculum and in its goals. Flexner spoke clearly and firmly, with minimal resort to indirection and between-the-lines messages. It is true, of course, that, unlike those who wrote the 1952 and 1953 reports, Flexner could count on the fact that there was a public readiness for what he recommended, that the most prestigious figures in the medical field were behind him, and that there would be money to start the change process. And, let us not forget, Flexner was not a physician, the foundation supporting his endeavor was not part of the medical establishment, and as a person—as his autobiography (1940) reveals—Flexner was forceful in a straitlaced, prophetic manner. It is, I think, fair to say that the impact of the 1910 report derives in part from the fact that a person and a foundation outside of medicine were responsible for the report. I am not being critical of the 1953 report when I characterize it as a conservative, indeed unimaginative document. The times were not conducive to a more radical report, because those were times when, as a result of the role of science and technology in World War II, the wedding that Flexner helped arrange between science and medicine was seen as not only fruitful but in its truly golden years. Psychiatry wanted to be seen as a legitimate offspring of that wedding. It was not disposed to criticize the house in which it wanted to live. Today it is even less disposed to do so, despite the fact that, for the first time since Flexner's report, the defects of medical education are getting nearer center stage of public and professional awareness.

What does the 1953 report recommend about how to achieve the goals of psychiatric training? Those goals are described as follows:

> The goal of a basic psychiatric training program is to develop, in adequately prepared physi-

cians, knowledge and understanding of mental
health and disease, and the skills and attitudes to
use such knowledge effectively in the care of patients and in the public interest. It is desirable also
that the resident develop the capacity to use his
knowledge and the community resources in community efforts for the preservation of mental
health; and that he develop interest in furthering
the progress of psychiatry through teaching and
research.

The resident's development is the chief objective of the training program. This involves the
growth of his capacity to assume and carry responsibility without being handicapped by his own anxiety; the practical use of his capacity for empathy,
responsiveness, and meaningful communication;
and the development of constructive attitudes
toward patients and their relatives, toward his colleagues and himself. Of major importance in the
resident's personal development are his relationships with key people of the training center faculty, their basic attitudes toward him, and the possibility of corrective emotional experience in the
learning process [American Psychiatric Association, 1953, p. 49].

Empathy, responsiveness, and meaningful communication—
these are not characteristics of an individual in the sense that
eye color, height, and weight are. They are concepts we invent
and use to characterize interactions between individuals. They
are normative judgments we make about what we see and hear
in interactions from which we infer what we think the participants think and feel. They are concepts about which there is
less than unanimity in regard to definition and even less agreement about whether in a particular interaction those concepts
are manifest in the clinician's behavior. If I prefer concepts such
as caring and compassion, it is not because I think they are better concepts but because they are more familiar to most people

and, in fact, are concepts more frequently used in current critiques of medical education (for example, Pellegrino, 1974).

In regard to psychiatric training, the 1953 report is unambiguous about the centrality of these concepts. There is a maxim that states that if you know how to select people, you have licked 50 percent of the problem of training them. The report is realistically pessimistic that customary procedures for selection have not been and will not be fruitful, and when that assessment is taken together with the adverse effects of the medical school experience on caring and compassionate behavior, it is clear that the problems in psychiatric training are formidable. The report is unambiguous about an additional, related assumption: caring and compassionate behavior requires an unusual degree of self-understanding that allows one to see commonalities between self and others. How can such self-understanding be attained? Here again, the report gives a clear general answer: the quality of clinical supervision. The supervisor, as the title denotes, has *super* vision that allows him or her to enable the supervisee to use the self as a vehicle for understanding others. Lectures, seminars, books, even sheer experience have their place, but, alone or in combination, they are no substitute for clinical supervision. Still, as any clinician will attest, supervisors vary considerably (to understate it somewhat) in what they consider the goals of supervision, the "technology" of supervision, the amount needed, and the emphasis on the relationship between the understanding of self and others. That a supervisor may be a superb clinician does not necessarily mean that he or she is an effective supervisor. The selection of supervisors presents the same issues as the selection of medical students and psychiatric trainees. But if I agree, as I do, that clinical supervision is the most effective means we have, that is not warrant for concluding that it is as effective as it should be in achieving its goals. If anything is clear in the training of any kind of clinician, it is that supervision is one of the least openly discussed and studied activities. The 1953 report does not illuminate these issues. To assume, as the report does, that clinical supervision is discernibly more than minimally effective in inculcating in the mind and behavior of the trainee the relationships between understanding self and others is understandable but not a source of satisfaction.

Training for the clinical endeavor does not take place in an institutional or societal vacuum. Although this is recognized by the 1953 report, that recognition has a dated quality in that it was written a decade before issues surrounding race, ethnicity, poverty, the distribution of health services, sexual orientation, the status of women, discrimination on the basis of handicap, and the needs of older people erupted into public awareness. Ours has always been a pluralistic society, but not until the late fifties was American medicine forced to begin to recognize how effectively it had insulated itself from that fact. That awakening had singular significance for psychiatry. Whereas psychiatrists had previously dealt with people more similar to than different from themselves—in interactions in which the relationship between understanding self and others was both central and problematic—they were not faced with types of people and issues that exposed the inadequacies of a course of training that ill prepared them for the changing scene. As never before, psychiatrists were criticized by these different "consumers" for a cultural parochialism that robbed them of the capacity to be caring and compassionate with those coming from backgrounds and life-styles foreign to the psychiatrist. Given the ambience of the sixties, it is not surprising that some of those entering psychiatry agreed with those criticisms, especially in regard to the redistribution of health services. They became activists and advocates, largely unaware of the possibility that, in advocating more of the same services for heretofore underserved populations, they might be exposing unwittingly the cultural parochialism from which they sought to unimprison themselves. That possibility aside, they were not disposed to recognize that, despite good intentions, they were faced with an exponential increase in the complexity of issues surrounding the understanding of self and others. Psychiatric training hardly changed at all, and, as I indicated earlier, it took just a few years for these sallies into the realities of the changing scene for psychiatry to revert to an emphasis on the biological basis and treatment of personal misery. For all practical purposes, the issues surrounding the understanding of self and others—certainly a central, if not *the* central issue in psychiatric training—became a cold, not a burning issue.

The 1953 report is not comprehensible unless an obvious feature of it is kept in mind: The stock-in-trade of the psychiatrist is knowledge and skills employed in a truly interpersonal encounter with someone in distress. Although the term *psychotherapy* is a generic one, encompassing differing theoretical orientations and styles, its distinguishing feature is the attempt by two people (sometimes more) to *understand each other,* to put into words thoughts and feelings that will be useful *to both* for purposes of action that will alleviate the personal distress about which one of them has sought help. To say that it is a sought-for interpersonal encounter is correct, but that characterization does not convey either the strength of feeling involved or the difficulties a clinician has in compassionately understanding the other person or (too frequently glossed over) the difficulties the client has in compassionately understanding the clinician. The report is unambiguous in stating that it is in the psychotherapeutic encounter that the centrality of caring and compassion to the clinical endeavor becomes manifest and, it is implied, to a degree that would not generally be found in other types of medical encounters. In light of the change in orientation that has taken place in psychiatry in recent years, it is justifiable to ask whether the use of drugs and the emphasis in training on biological treatment have had adverse effects on the caring and compassionate behavior of psychiatrists.

Let us pursue this possibility by way of an imaginary study. Suppose that it was possible on a particular day to videotape a random sample of interactions between psychiatrists and patients in the diverse settings in which these clinicians work: private office, outpatient clinic, general hospital, private psychiatric hospital, and state and VA hospitals. Let us also suppose that on that same day we can videotape interactions between patients and other medical specialists wherever they are at work. And let us assume that agreement has been reached about a set of reliable criteria by which a panel of professional and lay people can rate the presence and degree of caring and compassionate behavior of the diverse clinicians. Because this is an imaginary study, let us also assume that we have randomly chosen in a stratified way so that we have equal numbers of newly minted clinicians, those with five years of experience, those with ten years, and so on. Certainly, the first prediction one would assess is that psychiatrists would differ dramatically from other medical specialists in the presence and degree of caring and compassionate behavior. But what if the difference, although significant in a statistical sense is by no means dramatic? And how should we judge that difference if the nonpsychiatric specialties turn out to be as low as current reports on medical education suggest? If the nonpsychiatric specialties are not far above a zero point for caring and compassionate behavior, then the finding that psychiatrists get higher ratings is not a source for satisfaction unless those ratings are dramatically higher than those in other specialties.

If my experience is any guide, I would predict that psychiatrists, as a group, would not get dramatically higher ratings, especially in those cases and settings where medication is part of the treatment or, as in the case of psychiatric hospitals, medication is the primary basis of treatment. I would also predict that among neither psychiatrists nor other medical groups would increasing years of experience be correlated with increasing caring and compassionate behavior. Undergirding these predictions is the belief that socialization today in medical schools and psychiatric residencies interferes with rather than facilitates acquiring and reinforcing caring and compassionate behavior. In making these predictions, I could, of course, be very wrong in my beliefs; I could be overgeneralizing from admittedly limited experience, and I could be criticized for oversimplifying very complex interactional phenomena. These would not be criticisms advanced by psychiatrists insofar as predictions of their colleagues in other medical specialties are concerned. Psychiatrists have long been critical of the psychological and interpersonal obtuseness of other medical specialties. But they would certainly assert that that obtuseness is very rare among psychiatrists. If I take a contrary position, it is less to indulge my own beliefs than to suggest that it is by no means self-evident that the processes by which individuals self-select themselves for a career in psychiatry, the criteria by which they are selected, and the content of their psychiatric training—all occurring within the culture of medical schools and hospitals—contribute to caring and compassionate behavior. It is far from self-evident.

We are not dealing with an issue about which we can afford to assume that there is no means-end problem, that the best of motives and the most virtuous of goals are guarantors that the means we employ are appropriate to both motives and goals. And, I must reiterate, the barrage of criticism today being directed at medical education in particular and physicians generally is a sufficient basis for not exempting psychiatry, which in recent years has become so biologically reductionistic in theory and drug dispensing in practice. What I have attempted to demonstrate in this chapter is that in the modern history of psychiatry there have been two major ways by which psychiatry has tried to deepen and broaden the relationship between understanding (self and others), on the one hand, and effective caring and compassionate behavior in the therapeutic situation, on the other hand. One way was to sensitize the psychiatrist to social science, especially in regard to the importance of social-cultural-ethnic and religious factors in their historical emergence and present-day contexts. The second way was by an emphasis, some would say an agonizing one, of the complex dynamics of the clinical interaction. Today, both ways are far from center stage in psychiatric training.

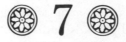

7

Clinical Psychology: New Profession, Old Answers

The issues surrounding caring and compassion in the provision of mental health services cannot be understood only by looking at a particular profession, such as psychiatry—that is, looking at it primarily in terms of how it selects and trains those who become part of it, or how it defines its role in society, or how tensions within it impede or facilitate change. Such a focus, albeit necessary and instructive, runs the risk of conveying the erroneous impression that the particular profession is, so to speak, captain of its fate and master of its soul. That impression, as the previous chapter indicated, is misleading in that psychiatry was not comprehensible unless one examined it in the context of American medicine generally and medical schools in particular. But that corrective is also, at best, partial, because neither American medicine nor psychiatry operates in outer space; they operate in a society with a distinctive history, traditions, and ideology. And it is not the case that you have two entities, psychiatry and society, affecting each other. If only by virtue of the fact that psychiatrists are socialized into the society, the profession is a reflection of that congery of variables subsumed under the concept of society. And precisely because society has legitimated the profession in diverse ways, it is a creation of the society.

How these complex transactions arise, develop, and change is fantastically complex, and it takes generations of scholars to unravel (a never-ending process) the nature and significance of the vicissitudes of those transactions. Matters are not helped any in this regard by the attitude, peculiarly but not uniquely American, that history is a museum of relics having no practical significance for present and future; that is, having no lineal descendants in the here and now. Nowhere is that attitude more apparent than in the mental health professions. It is true that in the 1952 report (American Psychiatric Association, 1952) discussed in the previous chapter there is recognition that, as a result of World War II, the world and American society would undergo momentous changes. What these changes might be, their strengths and conflict-producing protentials, their relationship to the near and far past—about such questions the report is quite silent, despite the stance that the society was changing. So, for example, the fact that the federal government, breaking with past traditions and practice, was becoming the major underwriter of mental health research, training, and clinical services was seen only as an unalloyed boon, not as a development that could be a mixed blessing, or one that had to be reviewed in light of the economic ups and downs that long characterized our society, or one that could have adverse effects on the profession as it wished to be. Far from examining these issues—if only because of the historically new relationship between psychiatry and government—the report looks to the future from an onward and upward stance, in this respect reflecting the stance of many people in the society. The war had been won, fascist tyranny had been vanquished, the United States had become the colossus of the world, science had helped win the war and would be the basis for sustaining a productive peace —the old world was dead, long live the new one!

If a new world was aborning, what might be some of its features, what of the old world would it contain, what might be some of the adverse consequences of the changes, and how might they be confronted? Granted that the new world would be dominated by scientific and technological developments—in ways and to a degree already demonstrated during World War II—on what basis could one assume that science and technology would be the universal solvents for the problematic momentous social changes that were already apparent and picking up steam? It is beyond the scope of this book to do justice to these questions, but there are certain parts of the answer that need to be briefly mentioned because of their relevance to how issues surrounding caring and compassion were virtually ignored by those in the mental health fields. Indeed, the exponential increase since World War II in the number and types of people providing mental health services to distressed individuals cannot be understood without addressing in brief some of these questions.

The end of World War II was greeted with hopes for and fantasies about a return to "normalcy": men and women, in and out of the armed forces, would return to their prewar jobs, to their neighborhoods and cities, to their nuclear and extended families, to "life" as they had known it. Yes, a new world was going to be built, but that new world would have many of the features of the old one. Call it the American Dream or the American Way of Life, the new world would be a "better" version. The desire "to return" existed side by side with the desire for change. And both desires were fed by outpourings of sheer relief that the frustrations, deprivations, loss of life, and carnage of war were at an end. It is not much of an exaggeration to say that many seemed to believe that the changes wrought by the war were reversible or, if not reversible, containable and remediable. These initial reactions to the end of the war were as unrealistic as they were understandable. Those who served in the armed services were changed forever, and families and spouses who lost loved ones were also changed as people. Most of those who returned home found that "you can't go home again," not only because of changes in the returnees but because those who remained at home had changed in diverse ways. And the society had changed in clear ways: women had become important in the workplace (and in the armed services), income levels had increased, life-styles (social and sexual) began discernibly to change, and there was anxiety about the economic threat that the discharge of millions of veterans represented to those who had remained in civilian life. And in the case of minorities, especially blacks returning to civilian life, they had no intention of accepting the discrimination that suffused "normalcy." They did not want to go home again! Let us not forget that the spurs to what were later called the civil rights and racial equality movements arose during World War II in the efforts to integrate the armed services. After all, you do not ask people to risk their lives in a war against Naziism and then expect them graciously to be victims of Nazi racist ideology. If during the war the armed services were far from communes of racial togetherness, they nevertheless altered the self-perceptions and expectations of blacks and other minorities.

One other feature of the war period requires emphasis: unprecedented geographical mobility. The severe labor shortage, the lure of increased income, and the attraction of urban areas where large defense plants had been built contributed to the growth and population diversity of urban areas, setting the stage of what in a few short years would become "the urban problem": racial and ethnic conflict and unrest, overburdened social services, rising juvenile delinquency rates, poverty, and accelerating ghettoization. If our cities looked different to returning veterans, so did the rural areas, which began to show the effects of loss of population.

There are real dangers in trying to sum up in a phrase or a few sentences a central theme intended to characterize the phenomenology of people at a particular time in a particular society when that society has all the features of a Bruegel painting: so much going on, overtly unrelated but covertly related, diverse types of people in almost every type of social and sexual relationship, so easy to miss the forest for the trees, so easy to want to close one's eyes to the bewildering array of frenzied movements. And when one discerns a central message, one knows (or should know) that one is distorting and narrowing the complexity, not because simplification is an inherent virtue but because language, however forceful and picturesque, is far from an adequate vehicle (albeit the best we have) for reflecting our vision. With that caveat, I shall now try to delineate aspects of the phenomenology of many people of the World War II era. I am not resorting to what C. Wright Mills called "psychologisms": trying to explain the social forces, structures, customs, traditions, and ideology of a society by resorting to an individual, asocial psychology, with the consequences of trivializing the concept of society and making individual behavior incomprehensible. And when, perforce, one makes the individual figure and the society background, it should always be for the moment, so to speak, to be replaced by a deliberate reversal of the figure-ground relationship. It is a bedeviling problem and process, which the mental health fields have hardly recognized.

Who am I? How have I changed? How will I have to change? Will I be able to adjust? Do I want to adjust? How do I make up for lost time? Where should I go to start over? Why do I feel strange with those who should not be strangers to me? Why do things look so different? How come things have changed so much? Why can't I explain to people what I experienced and what it meant to me? Why are they so much more interested in their future than in my past? These are questions that millions of veterans asked, but each of them had its counterpart in the phenomenology of friends and families of the returnees. Almost everything and everybody had changed, not least those who had remained in civilian life, usually unaware that they had changed in a changing society at war.

People felt, almost palpably, a discontinuity with their past, a sense of strangeness with self, an unease about the future. The bonds that interconnect people within the family, among friends, in the neighborhood, and in the work site had languished. These bonds often may be mixed blessings, but bonds they are, reflecting structure, predictability, and obligation. They are bonds that define self, others, and the world. But when those bonds go by the boards, whatever the reasons, people feel at sea. The sense of discontinuity and lack of bondedness spurred many people to seek a geographical change of scene, and the migration westward, particularly to California, noticeably increased, further and farther separating people from their prewar origins.

Another way of putting what I have said is that the ending of the war and its immediate aftermath engendered in large segments of society a reaction of surprise: they and the world that shaped them had certainly and irrevocably changed, and there was to be no return to "normalcy." There were those, of course, who knew that a return to "normalcy" would be a return to disaster. The Great Depression was part of the prologue of World War II and had incalculable and lasting effects, some of which were not diluted in strength until our country began to gear up to cope with the fascist dictatorships. Indeed, the memory of the Great Depression—responsible in its own way for changing life-styles and family roles and cohesion, for migration from one part of the country to another, for a sense of discontinuity with the past and a resignation to a dark future, and for the sense that one lived in an uncaring, uncompassionate world—that memory was still fresh in people's minds at the end of World War II and was the basis of the fear that, with the return of millions of veterans to civilian life, the country again would be plunged into economic chaos and social unrest. It was a memory, indeed a specter, that haunted political leaders and played a significant role in legislation (for example, the Full Employment Practices Act of 1946 and the GI Bill of Rights, about which more in a little while).

Elsewhere (Sarason, 1977), in discussing those years, I have said that World War II ushered in the age of psychology or the age of mental health. And in applying those designations, I was trying to convey several things. First, the thirties and forties, for different but related reasons, forced people to look inward, to be preoccupied with self. In the thirties, with at least 20 percent of the population unemployed, the questions were: Will I (we) survive economically, will I go hungry, will I ever work again? In the war period, the questions for someone in the armed forces (and their loved ones) were: Will I break down, will I be injured? Try living with questions like that for several years without concern for your psychological stability. No doubt that some people grow in adversity: no doubt far more are disabled by sustained adversities. The second point was that, in the thirties and forties, again for different but related reasons, the stability of family relationships was markedly weakened and subject to stress, and this would show up, generally speaking, in psychological symptomatology in adjacent generations. This did not mean that people were "going to pieces" but rather that there was an increasing awareness of the private sense that one did not understand self or others; that is, that one sought explanations of that sense of aloneness, of alienation from self and others, for directions for how to make "sense and contact." In a world that was increasingly secular and did not provide satisfying explanations for one's questions and plight, many individuals felt like a snowflake in a storm. What I am describing is not a new kind of consciousness in Western society; it had a long history. But World War II drastically accelerated this emerging world view, vitiating many of the bonds that gave purpose to one's life and social relationships.

World War II was a long war. We entered the war December 7, 1941, but the draft had begun two years before. With the beginning of the draft and then our entry into the war, the public was forced to become aware of casualties, physical and psychological. As I indicated in an earlier chapter, it was immediately apparent that as a society we were and would be faced, on an unprecedented scale, with individuals incapacitated by personal misery and disorder. In one sense, it is correct to say that the scale of the problem within the armed services, and then the problems of "normal" returnees to civilian life, triggered public sensitivity to psychology as a vehicle for comprehending self and others. But, in another sense, it is misleading, because it ignores or underemphasizes how ready people in general were for a psychology that was both explanation and salvation. It was a readiness that was subliminal, waiting, so to speak, for changes in the larger society to give it manifest expression. And World War II contained and stimulated those changes. If psychiatry, psychology, and other mental health professions seized the opportunity to promote their services, orientation, and recommendations—and, let us not forget, their representatives were already in the corridors of the federal government and the offices of planning and policy—their success said far less about their entrepreneurship than it did about the readiness of the larger society to hear their message. Unfortunately, it was a message to and about individuals, not about the forces and contexts that had rendered individual existence so problematic. It offered a personal service for what was a manifestation of complex social change. It offered caring and compassion on an individual basis, as if that would be adequate to contain and ameliorate the ongoing consequences of fragile, unsatisfying social and family bonds. And if a lot was promised, if caring and compassion were central to a service to be purchased for a fee, it did not extend much beyond those who were white, educated, urban, and middle class.

The point I am making here is that the mental health professions seemed unaware that, in recognizing the need in people from backgrounds similar to their own for a caring and compassionate relationship with a psychotherapist, they were, for all practical purposes, uncaring and uncompassionate toward large segments of the population who had, for many of the same reasons, the same need for caring, compassionate psychological help. This, of course, is not to say that mental health personnel were, as individuals, uncaring and uncompassionate but rather that they had the most narrow and incomplete understanding of how and why the society had changed and would continue to change. And there was unintended wisdom in this narrowness, because, if their understanding had been more broad, they would have to have faced then what they were forced to face two decades later: that their dominant theories of individual behavior and the helping process, and the role and nature of caring and compassion in that process, were very inadequate when extended to groups who differed radically from the professional in terms of race, ethnicity, education, and economic status. And, as the emerging women's liberation movement began to indicate and criticize, the male-dominated mental health professions, based as they were on rampantly prejudiced views of women and their place in the home and in work, could not be caring and compassionate about the plight of women. How could they be other than superficially caring and compassionate when their training and theories rendered them blind to the problem? How could professionals trained to rivet on the intrapsychic workings of the individual mind become sensitive to how the social world viewed and acted toward women in accordance with the dynamics of the self-fulfilling prophecy? Infinitely more than any of the mental health professions, from early on, the different group movements clearly saw that there were wide gulfs between the givers and recipients of care and compassion. Caring and compassion are not characteristics of an individual but ascriptions to interactions where the goal is to overcome the barriers, societally engendered and sustained, to mutual understanding.

A final note on the years immediately following the war. It concerns one of the truly momentous and change-producing legislative acts of this century: the GI Bill of Rights. I am not concerned here with the considerations that led to that legislation. For my purposes, its significance lies in the fact that the legislation literally underwrote the opportunity for millions of individuals to alter the course of their lives, to aspire to goals that had been unrealistic for them before the war, to become different kinds of people than their backgrounds would ordinarily have allowed, and, for an undetermined but not small number of people, to have the time to figure out who they were, what they might become, how to deal effectively with the discontinuities engendered in them by the war. What the GI Bill meant was that individuals who had already experienced significant personal change would experience even more change. And for many (not all) of these veterans, it meant still another geographical change in living site, more psychological distance from their backgrounds, another postponement of that sought-for feeling of interpersonal and vocational permanence. From one standpoint, the GI Bill was an unrivaled boon provided by a grateful society somewhat fearful of what could happen if millions of veterans were catapulted back into society without purpose and support. As a result of that bill, counseling centers were developed (it seemed) overnight and everywhere. Anyone who was on the staff of one of those centers will attest to two things: the wisdom in passing that legislation and the bewilderment of many veterans at the "Who am I, what should I be, can I be?" problem.

It is hard to convey to the younger reader how crowded (again, almost overnight) our colleges and universities became, with row upon row of Quonset huts used for living, teaching, and administering. To what areas of concentration were under-graduate and graduate students attracted? Before World War II, the number of undergraduate majors in psychology was not re-markable, and the number seeking their doctorate in that field was also unremarkable. Within very few years after the war—only two years, if my memory is correct—the number who took psychology as an undergraduate major or sought to enter a doc-toral program began to escalate. This was true for both veterans and nonveterans, and that escalation did not cease until the mid-seventies. Psychology departments grew, some in our state universities becoming enormous, because the demand for psy-chology courses seemed insatiable. There is no simple explana-tion for this dramatic switch, but there can be no doubt that psychology symbolized something that spoke directly to what people thought they needed. I do not think I am resorting to hyperbole when I suggest that psychology—as a body of knowl-edge, as a means for self-understanding, as a compass for living—had taken on some of the features of tradition and religion. It was the secular answer to the questions: What is humanity? How do we justify an existence? How should we live with each other? How do we define good and bad, virtue and sin?

If the significance of the emerging age of psychology was not understood, let alone confronted, by psychiatry, it was a re-flection of the fact that psychiatry was a clinical discipline: it dealt with the problems of individuals that already existed and sought to alleviate individual personal distress, and neither by tradition nor by theoretical orientation could it focus other than superficially on the larger social picture in which these problems were embedded. I am quite aware that the years I have so briefly described were not easy to fathom or analyze, and I am not one who believes that the present is pregnant with only one future. But two features of those years were clear: the sense that vast social changes had occurred and would continue to occur—not only in this country but in the world at large—and the sense that the bonds that hold together the structure of and give meaning to individual existence and the societal fabric had been dramatically weakened. Precisely because it rivets atten-tion on the problems of individuals, the clinical endeavor is, for all practical purposes, rendered impotent to see the larger picture and, therefore, to assess how its ways of providing services, and to whom, might be altered in substance and goals.

Let us turn now to another profession, clinical psychology, which was, so to speak, born in the years immediately following World War II. That profession, which grew like Topsy in subsequent decades, is instructive in a number of ways. First, for all practical purposes, there was no profession of clinical psychology in prewar psychology; that is, training for such a professional activity simply was not available in departments of psychology. Second, unlike psychiatry, psychology had been primarily a social science. Third, in forging a new and modern clinical discipline, psychology very self-consciously was responding to a perceived societal need for new knowledge and improved clinical practice. Fourth, because of its strong scientific, research, and experimental ideology and traditions, the possibility existed that the new clinical discipline could move the mental health area in new directions. Fifth, from its very beginnings, many of its founders wished to discourage the private practice of clinical psychology; that is, they felt that the need for clinicians in public agencies and institutions should take priority over private practice. Finally, the creation and meteoric growth of clinical psychology were among the telling indicators of the age of psychology. Reflecting on the growth of the American Psychological Association—which in the postwar period has grown from a few thousand to over sixty thousand members (not all clinical psychologists, of course)—someone wryly pointed out that, if the trend continued, there would in the year 2000 be more psychologists than people.

So what happened? In order to answer that question, you have to read carefully *Training in Clinical Psychology* (Raimy, 1950), a report of a two-week conference in 1949 attended by seventy-one representatives from universities, mental health service agencies, and allied professions. I attended that "founding" conference (known as the Boulder conference). It was an amazingly serious, well organized, and yet intellectually freewheeling conference that, like the Flexner report, shaped the future of a field. The critique I now offer is in its essentials similar to the position I took at the conference, a position I argued for vigorously and unsuccessfully. I do not wish to convey the impression that the points I raised were as clear in my head then as I think they are now. At that time, I was only beginning to become aware that American psychology, far from taking social contexts seriously and erasing arbitrary boundaries between it and other social sciences, was a psychology of the asocial, isolated individual. Although social psychology had always been a major field in psychology, the relation between *social* and *societal* was much more linguistic than conceptual. So, for example, you can read all 253 pages of the report and not get the faintest idea of what was happening in the society at the time. In that respect, in comparison to the Flexner report, the Boulder report and the one in psychiatry three years later (American Psychiatric Association, 1953, discussed in the previous chapter) were glaringly deficient. They seemed to assume that there was no relevant history to ponder, that ours was a homogeneous society, that psychologists were a random sample of the population, that the world view of psychologists was based only on purity of spirit and nobility of purpose, that one did not have to fear that well-intentioned professionalism might get converted to self-serving guildism, that the universe of alternatives the new field might take was narrow, that the history of American medicine and psychiatry was devoid of significance for the new clinical discipline, and, perhaps most troublesome of all, that this new discipline could ally itself, as it very deliberately sought to do, with psychiatry and the medical setting without getting caught up in their imperialistic, competitive institutional ambience and without taking on the major problematic features of their training practices. The reader who has doubts on this score, especially in regard to training, should scrutinize the contents of the training program contained in the report. In spirit, content, and purpose, it has affinity to the Flexner report, which is never mentioned in the report of the Boulder conference.

The position I took at the Boulder conference did not derive from a superior knowledge of the history of the issues or of professionalism in American society or from any unusual clarity about what the future held in store. My position had two sources. The first was the year of training I spent in a state psychiatric hospital, during which I never felt that I understood or was helped to understand patients as persons. It was small balm that the psychiatrists, who literally controlled and ran the institution, did not seem disposed to see patients other than through the prism of theories, abstractions, and jargon. They were no less caring and compassionate than I was—callous youth that I was, they may have been more caring and compassionate than I —but I could see little or nothing to suggest that in their relationships with patients they saw them other than as a collection of symptoms. I have no doubt that every member of the professional staff had read and been moved by Clifford Beers's description of what it was like to be a patient in the uncomprehending world of the psychiatric hospital.

It would be grossly incorrect and unfair to say that Worcester State Hospital was like the one described in *One Flew Over the Cuckoo's Nest* or like the hospitals described by Albert Deutsch (1948) in his *The Shame of the States*. Indeed, when I was at Worcester State Hospital in 1941-42, it was regarded as the best in the country in terms of quality of staff and administration (in psychiatry and psychology), quality of training, and quality of its research programs in the biology and treatment of mental disorders. It is safe to say that, between 1935 and 1942, that hospital contributed as many (if not more) leaders to academic psychiatry and clinical psychology in the post–World War II era as all of the country's other state hospitals combined. I learned many things, but how to understand patients as persons was not one of them. There is a maxim in public education that says that you teach children, not subject matter. What I learned at Worcester was how easy it was (and still is) to treat diagnostic categories rather than people. I also learned how in the psychiatric setting—in any complex setting for human service—the needs of the staff unwittingly but insidiously come to take precedence over the needs of those the setting is designed to serve. And if I learned anything in the psychiatric setting, it was how little time the professional staff spent with patients, in which respect Worcester was no different from any other hospital. It was caring and compassionate behavior on the run, so to speak.

The second source of the position I took at the Boulder conference was the several years I spent as a clinical psychologist at the Southbury State Training School for mentally retarded people, a post I accepted, in preference to two others in psychiatric hospitals, with eagerness and enthusiasm, feelings that friends and others found difficult to comprehend. Why on earth would anyone *choose* to work with mentally retarded individuals, who were uninteresting, from whom one could expect only slow and limited improvement, many of whom looked odd (ugly), and who lacked an "inner" life? If such a choice was strange, it was even more strange to others that I *enjoyed* being with, relating to, trying to understand those people (they were called children then; they were human, of course, but that label represented more an act of charity than any ascription of meaningful affinity). I chose to take this position not because I was eager to work with this population but because it was a new institution, with an explicit nonmedical, educational purpose, and I would have freedom to do pretty much what I wanted to do. As it turned out, I quickly came to see these people as persons, each in his or her own way concerned with problems in living: separation from family, desire for psychological and physical intimacy, curiosity about the purposes of others, and so on. By the time I left Southbury to go to Yale, I could no longer think of these people as mentally retarded; that is, as members of a diagnostic category sharing characteristics associated with that category. Each was a distinctive individual.

What the experience at Southbury taught me is how insidiously easy and unwitting it is to see people from the perspective of clinical categories, thus effectively interfering with those processes of understanding that make caring and compassionate behavior possible. A concrete example: if your neighbor's child, who has an IQ of 180, takes your cat and crushes it to death, you will not say he did it *because* he has an IQ of 180. But if your neighbor's child has an IQ of 60, you very likely would invoke in your explanation the low IQ as the etiological agent without which the event would not have occurred. The willingness to seek to understand another person with the seriousness you would want someone to seek to understand you, in the kinds of terms that interrelate one's private and public, covert and overt behavior, makes it likely that caring and compassion will follow. At the Boulder conference, I resented the fact that it was recommending a direction that would make it unlikely that clinical psychologists would ever work with mentally retarded individuals. I resented even more the attitude that this population was uninteresting, undeserving of the attention of this new clinical discipline. What I did not see clearly then was that this new clinical field was shutting itself off from working with diverse groups and segments of the society, not on the basis of principle or of some process of "thinking through" but on the basis of what were then familiar clinical problems and issues the study and treatment of which federal funding agencies had made clear they wished to support. There was no seduction involved; there was no conflict whatsoever between the intentions of the representatives from the government and those of the universities.

Everyone at the Boulder conference knew that there was a vast discrepancy between the number of trained clinicians (psychological and psychiatric) and the number of people who wished to use their services and that that discrepancy would probably grow with the years. How do we justify a strategy that in practice means that clinicians would not have experience with anything resembling a representative sample of this heterogeneous society? On what basis do we assume that our knowledge of clinical training is sufficiently solid and our methods sufficiently effective as to ensure that, despite restriction in the kinds of people served, that training will permit the clinician to be understanding, caring, and compassionate when individuals from unfamiliar backgrounds are encountered? Is caring and compassionate behavior something you learn and, having learned it, you never have to learn again, regardless of who seeks your help? Embarked as we are on forging a new clinical discipline, should we not, consistent with the experimental traditions of American psychology, experiment with criteria for selection and modes of training? Is there any basis for complacency about the efficiency of current modes of training for understanding self and others? Unfortunately, these questions were not raised or seriously discussed at the Boulder conference. In fact, almost every criticism I advanced in the previous chapter about the 1953 report on psychiatric training applies to the Boulder report, and, I must add, with more justification, because psychology had long considered itself a part of the social sciences and therefore, presumably, more sensitive to the diversity of groups, cultures, and classes so obvious a feature of American society.

I have raised two different but in practice highly interconnected issues. The first has to do with how self-consciously a clinical discipline apportions its resources in light of the obvious diversity of populations the society contains. The second is how sensitive the discipline is to the special obligations that diversity places on training for understanding when clinician and client vary considerably in age, background, ethnicity, race, social class, and so on. After all, what is distinctive, if not unique, in the clinical endeavor in the mental health fields is the quest for understanding people as complex persons, and if that understanding is narrow, or wrong, or distorted, the stage is set for these clinicians to be seen as uncaring and uncompassionate. Any conception of the helping process that is not based on a conception of the nature of our complex society and how it intrudes directly and inevitably into the clinical-client interaction automatically restricts the achievement of that process's therapeutic objectives. The degree of that restriction became obvious in the turbulent sixties, when blacks, gays, diverse ethnic groups, handicapped people, young and old people, and women called into question the orientation and practices of the mental health professions. And by calling into question I mean that they saw these clinicians as well-meaning, parochial people whose theories and practices rendered them unfit to comprehend their plight.

An egregious example: For at least fifteen years after World War II, the Veterans Administration underwrote the graduate education and clinical training of more clinical psychologists than any other agency (or any several combined). In fact, the VA sponsored and in large part underwrote the Boulder conference, because it had such a stake in getting clinical psychologists for staff positions. That meant that the clinical training had to (literally) take place in VA hospitals and clinics, and that meant that the clinical trainees would never see children and would very rarely see women. It is true but too easy to say that this can be explained primarily by the financial incentives the VA dangled before students and graduate departments of psychology. Underlying these contractual arrangements was an assumption as invalid as it was unarticulate: that the training the student would get for understanding human behavior and the helping process would be transferable to populations radically different from those encountered in VA facilities. This assumption is redolent of the position held much earlier in this century that exposure to mathematics or to Latin (preferably to both) instills a clarity of thinking and precision in logic that will be generalized elsewhere in a student's experience. It took a while for that assumption to be invalidated by American psychology. It is ironic that when, after World War II, issues surrounding the training of clinical psychologists came to the fore, that assumption was unreflectively accepted. Understanding, caring, and compassion—qualities of the clinical interaction that no one questioned (or questions)—were seen as almost platonic essences in the clinician that would become manifest regardless of the kinds of social gulfs that would exist between clinician and client, regardless of the restricted range of clients to which the student would be exposed.

In regard to restricted range of training experience, I must make brief mention here of another factor, to which I shall return in a later chapter. It is one of those factors that are obvious but whose implications have not been seriously explored and their significances for selection and training have hardly taken into account. I refer to the fact that the bulk of people who seek and are selected for a career in psychiatry and clinical psychology are young and have spent the years between early childhood and adulthood in settings clearly restrictive of range of experience. I am not talking here about personal maturity, however defined, and the role it plays in understanding others. It is to the credit of the 1953 report on the training of psychiatrists that it finds the extent of personal immaturity among medical students and psychiatric residents worrisome. The Boulder report is strangely silent on this score, although my experience in the training of clinical psychologists certainly confirms what the 1953 report says. The point I wish to emphasize here can be put in the form of an assumption: to a certain extent, at least, range of experience in the "real world" facilitates that kind of understanding of others that makes for caring and compassionate behavior. Albeit indirectly, that assumption is in principle one that has long undergirded the argument for a liberal education: that one is not "liberated" from intellectual narrowness, imprisoning cultural parochialisms, the impoverishments of the ahistorical stance, the mindless rejection of tradition, without serious exposure to the diverse ways people have sought and continue to seek understanding of themselves and their world.

Beginning with Flexner in 1910 and right up through the years to today, the liberal arts curriculum has been viewed as a kind of insurance against the constraints of later specialization in clinical fields, not the least of which are the pressures that underly and narrow one's social perspectives and obligations. The objectives of that curriculum, which for long were prescribed, were to be achieved in the setting of the college and university—broad objectives in a socially and physically restricted setting. If these objectives were never fully met—if the lack of concomitant broadening experience in the larger society set limits to what could be learned in and generalized from the college classroom—the pursuit of these objectives was more than a token gesture to the principle of the broadening of horizons. It certainly was not a token gesture on Flexner's part when he briefly but stirringly asserted that a liberal arts education was the best and only way to ensure that the future physician would attain "the requisite insight and sympathy" without which sensitivity to needs and plights of others is absent. But it soon became a token gesture as the premedical curriculum centered around science and technology, an emphasis that vastly accelerated after World War II, despite the fact that the reports on the training of psychiatrists and clinical psychologists contain clear warnings about the baleful effects of such emphasis.

That those who seek careers in clinical fields have a narrow range of experience has to be seen in relation to the additional fact that they are, as a group, the opposite of a random selection from the general population in terms of race, gender, social class, and religious affiliation. It is true that in recent decades the barriers to the admission of women have been dramatically weakened, but those who are admitted are in other respects no different from men. We cannot, of course, say what the changes, if any, will be over the long run by elimination of these barriers. For over four decades, I have participated in the training of clinical psychologists, and in the past fifteen years that has meant working with many young women. In regard to such factors as range of cultural and vocational experiences and breadth of undergraduate education, I have discerned no differences between women and men. And in terms of the obstacles these limitations present in the clinical training of these young people, men and women differ not at all. That men and women clinical students differ in many respects I do not question, but, whatever those differences, they do not withstand the pressures for socialization into the profession. And in the post-World War II era, those pressures—which had infiltrated into the college and school years—have exacerbated rather than compensated for narrowness of experience and understanding. That is not my conclusion alone. Students thirst for diversity of experience; they are quite aware of how narrow their experiences have been; they are frequently overwhelmed by their inability to understand others for whom they have a responsibility; they are often troubled by having to learn to suppress spontaneous feeling and action, which, they are told, are inimical to the clinical role; and many of them resent the process by which they are being shaped to fit a predetermined, narrow professional role. Far more than some of their mentors, many students are agonizingly aware of how impoverished their educational and social-cultural experiences have been for the task of understanding and caring for others. As a student once said to me, "I am learning *to act* as if I understand and care. I *do* care, but I rarely feel I *understand.* And most of the time I end up with a lot of unexpressed caring that is unrelated to my acting."

In light of these considerations, it should occasion no surprise that in the reports on the training of clinical psychologists and psychiatrists, as in the Flexner report, the concept of supervision is central. What should occasion surprise is the generality and vagueness with which the concept is discussed. In part, this is because the need for and the goals of supervision are deemed self-evident: for the protection of the client as well as for the needs of the young, developing professional, the clinical interaction has to be gone over (or prepared for) with someone with *super* vision and *super* understanding of the interconnections among understanding, caring, and compassion. The goal is never technical in a narrow sense; it is always to enlarge understanding of self and others, which will then serve as a basis for compassionate actions. But how does one help the prospective clinician gain enlarged understanding of another person? How does one help the student see how his or her limitations of experience affect understanding of others? If, as no one has ever denied, the student's very real limitations of knowledge and experience have to be confronted and overcome, then these limitations have to be as much in the focus of the supervision as the problems of the client. And those limitations, again as no one has ever denied, are narrowness of personal experience; of knowledge of and contact with cultural, racial, and social class groupings; of educational and intellectual horizons; and of conceptions of the change process. As a clinical colleague once said: "You can never go wrong overestimating the ignorance of trainees." And as I and many other supervisors will say: "Our most egregious errors derived from underestimating the limitations of trainees."

The goals of supervision are, in principle, awesome, because they require the forging of conceptual connections between a particular trainee and a particular patient, both of whom, as individuals and as a dyad, are reflections of an amazingly heterogeneous society of which they are members and products. To the extent that supervision focuses primarily on the client, or on narrow, technical, procedural matters, or on illustrating and following a particular theory of therapy, supervision becomes far less awesome. It also becomes far less of a liberating experience for the student, and by liberating I mean freeing one from the confines of a parochial view of the social world in which one lives.

An example: A student was presenting to me his first psychotherapeutic session with a man who was fifty-five years of age, an immigrant from a central European country, and a teacher of history in a private school. There were problems in his childless marriage, and it was not clear whether he was coming voluntarily or as a result of pressure from his wife. The student described the patient as overcontrolled, respectful, somewhat imperious in manner, and seemingly uncomfortable about what he should say and when. Early in the hour, he asked the student: "What is psychotherapy?" The student did not answer the question but instead asked: "Why do you ask that question?" The man was obviously dissatisfied with the student but politely said that he had asked the question because he was frankly puzzled about what psychotherapy was and how it worked. To which the student replied: "You will get an understanding as we continue to meet."

The student's attitude and gambit did not surprise me, because it is by no means unusual for beginners to hold to a picture of the psychotherapist as someone who passively listens, who nonverbally conveys sincere interest and compassion, who makes wise interpretations every now and then, and who never falls into the "trap" of directly answering a direct question. It is the popular picture of the analyst behind the couch. In vigorously pursuing why the student did not answer the question, I was interested in far more than how the student justified his lack of response, because I assumed—correctly, it turned out—that he would say that the question the man put to him was a defense against talking about his problems; that is, that he preferred an intellectual discussion to a personally revealing one. How, I asked, did you know fifteen minutes into the first hour that this was a defense? And what if it was a defense? Does that mean that you never answer a question that reflects a defensive maneuver? What one should do, the student said, is to inter-pret, not answer, such questions. What, I asked, would you have done if in this hour, during which you felt that he was quite anxious, he had asked you where the toilet is? Would you have refused to tell him because you were convinced that he wanted time out from you? The student agreed that he would tell him where the toilet is, because he understood from his own experi-ence the relationship between anxiety and urination and defeca-tion.

If I had stopped at this point, I would have felt that I had done the student a service, but within narrow, albeit important, limits. No less important than the issues surrounding answering a client's questions were those deriving from two indisputable differences between student and patient. The first was that the student was twenty-three and the man fifty-five years of age. How, I asked the student, do you think Mr. X interpreted the significance of the fact that he was a good deal older than you? That question had not occurred to the student, even though the student was aware that Mr. X was much older than he. If the student was aware of the age difference, was it not likely that Mr. X was? The student agreed that was likely the case. Granted, I went on, that not all men of Mr. X's age would react in the same way, would there not be some commonalities in re-gard to how distraught fifty-five-year-old men would feel about being personally revealing to a twenty-three-year-old male? Is ours a society that downplays age segregation, that makes older people feel worthy and wanted, that makes it easy for males to age with grace? Is it not likely that men of this age will call their masculinity into question, because, in our society, masculinity and dependency are antitheses? And is it not likely, I went on, that the refusal to answer his question was adding insult to an already injured male ego?

I could go on and on (as I frequently do with students), but the point is that this student had been unable to see the in-teraction as an instance of how features of the larger society infiltrate into the clinical endeavor. This was not due to per-sonal immaturity or blind spots in the student's makeup. And it certainly was not because he was incapable of being compassionate. He lacked the range of experience that might have sensitized him to the ways in which age and aging characterize myriad relationships in our society. It was not that the student had not been in situations analogous to the one Mr. X found himself in. After all, his relationship with me was pervaded by both of us being sensitive to a wide age difference. Neither his formal education nor social living had given him a basis, however superficial, for understanding how age is a ubiquitous factor in human relationships, its manifestations varying considerably within our society and between ours and other societies. And lacking that understanding, he was not, in my opinion, appropriately caring and compassionate. Quite the opposite.

The second indisputable difference was that the student was born and reared in this country and Mr. X had spent the first forty years of his life in a central European country. In hearing the description of Mr. X, I could not avoid the impression that Mr. X was like some Europeans who had been very important in my life. They derogated American society, saw it on a downhill course, and viewed it as self-defeatingly tolerant of waste, laziness, and wishy-washy discipline. Mr. X's appearance had a Prussian-like quality. When I told the student what got conjured up in my mind, he thought I had got the picture he intended me to get. In that event, as I had learned about my friends, one had to be sensitive to what it meant to Mr. X to leave his country of birth (at age forty) and resettle in a strange, bewilderingly diverse country. He and his wife had very few friends, and they also tended to have come from the home country. I said all this and more to the student, emphasizing the possibility that Mr. X's social bearing in the hour was in part a reflection of what can happen when one moves from one society to another; one does not want to appear strange, different, and inferior, yet at the same time one is plagued by just those feelings. Whatever Mr. X's presenting problem, it could not, I assumed, be unrelated to the single most important event in his life: leaving his home country to live forever in a new one. And, I continued, when Mr. X asked what psychotherapy was, there was a way of understanding him that would have played down the defensive feature of the question and would have given the benefit of the doubt to the possibility that Mr. X has never been part of the age of psychology. The question Mr. X asked was understood by the student in terms of the dynamics of the here and now. What the student did not understand, what I do not expect students to know except as a disembodied abstraction, is that the here and now has a seamless boundary with a vast, continuous, psychological, and sociocultural past. Without that understanding, caring and compassion are likely to be misdirected and ineffective. I told the student that I would not be surprised if Mr. X did not return for the next session. He did not return. I instructed the student to call him up to request that he come in because he wanted to explain the nature of psychotherapy. Mr. X returned and the relationship was resumed. If anything was clear from the subsequent sessions, it was that Mr. X did not grow up in the American age of psychology.

If you view the goal of supervision to be the broadening of perspectives about people in and of a society, it is a time-consuming affair. That is the case even if the goal is limited to narrow psychological considerations. As I said earlier, no one, at least on a verbal level, denies the crucial significance of supervision in the training of any kind of clinician. However, one might not discern this from observation of customary practice. For example, in medical training, it is usually the case that the student or intern-resident receives the bulk of supervision from someone a notch or two above the student's level of experience. If this is not a case of "in the land of the blind, the one-eyed man is king," it certainly approaches it. This practice is less frequent but by no means rare in the training of mental health clinicians. In all of these instances, the proffered rationale starts with the recognition that supervision is a very serious and time-consuming affair, then states that those with *super* vision are too few in number and trainees too many in number to handle the situation, and concludes with the argument that, if relatively inexperienced clinicians are to learn about supervision, they have to begin sometime. Someone once said that this is a conception of quality control that clinicians would not willingly accept in regard to other human endeavors. There are those who would argue that these practices, by and large, "work." Indeed,

they do work, but in a superficial, non-Jamesian conception of
the pragmatic. Pragmatism emphasizes the contemplation,
analysis, and evaluation of the consequences of actions in relation to the purposes or goals of those actions. Consequences are
meaningless, or at best mischievously misleading, independent
of their relation to stated purposes. When it is said that the
supervisory practice works, it is in relation to extraordinarily
narrow purposes primarily technical in substance and range. If
there is mounting dissatisfaction with those in the clinical endeavor, it is in part because of the failure to examine critically
the goals of supervision and to avoid the trap of transforming
educational into technical goals.

The clinical endeavor is quintessentially social in two
senses: it involves two people seeking to understand each other,
and it is an interaction that in myriad ways bears the imprint of
important features of the society. It may involve technical
knowledge and procedures, but they are always means for
understanding and helping. (Let us not forget that the clinician
seeks the patient's help no less than the patient seeks the clinician's help.) Supervision of the prospective clinician that does
not take seriously the social in these two senses—that does not
broaden the student's conception of self, others, and the society
—limits the degree to which that student will be appropriately
caring and compassionate. And I say *appropriately* to emphasize
that the issue is not whether the clinician wants to be compassionate but whether his or her actions are experienced by the
other person as compassionate. I have never met a clinician who
did not regard him- or herself as compassionate, a fact that does
not explain why so many people see some clinicians as otherwise.

In their organizational forms, be it in a university or in
professional society, professions have never been noted for their
capacity to scrutinize and evaluate the process by which they
admit and socialize people into their field. This is not to say, of
course, that they are unconcerned about these matters. That
would be grossly untrue and unfair. But it is neither unfair nor
untrue to say that the clinical professions have done surprisingly
little to determine the degree to which the people they admit

and train meet standards of caring and compassion. Every now and then, as I indicated in earlier chapters, individuals or some small group articulate their concerns in unvarnished language to which, to my knowledge, no one has attempted a rebuttal. In part, the lack of reaction (let alone change) may be due to the anecdotal nature of the data upon which these concerns rest. A major reason Flexner's report had impact is that he not only visited every medical school in this country and Canada but described in detail and dispassionately what he saw. No reader of that report was left in doubt about what went on in medical training, what passed for clinical and laboratory facilities, and how well students were prepared to engage in medical practice. And when Flexner concluded by damning the bulk of these schools, few were foolish enough to argue with him.

Insofar as caring and compassionate behavior of clinicians is concerned, there has been very little research, and what there is is no source for comfort. This is surprising when one considers the extent to which, in the post–World War II period, the clinical fields sought and received ever-increasing support for research. One would think that research on the efficacy of training would have been vigorously pursued, that the effort to improve the quality of the clinical endeavor through research would have included a focus on the behavior of clinicians. That has not been the case. It is as if virtuous intentions—presumably self-evidently present in teacher and student—are deemed sufficient to achieve the goal of producing caring and compassionate clinicians. Somewhere in biblical writings is the admonition that you will be judged not by what is in your heart but by what you do. It is an admonition that the clinical fields have yet to take seriously.

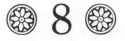

8

Behind
and Beyond Labels

Labels are necessary linguistic inventions that too frequently and effectively obscure commonalities among roles and activities that have different labels. So, when we hear the label *clinical,* the imagery conjured up in our minds is of physicians, clinics, and hospitals, of sick people seeking help from specially trained medical and allied personnel. We do not think of teachers and lawyers as clinicians. Those labels conjure up imagery not tied to medical settings, and, therefore, we are unable to see in what ways teachers, lawyers, and physicians essentially can be in similar roles. We begin to see these similarities, and then only vaguely and intuitively, when societal and institutional changes call into question the efficacy of those performing these clinical functions. This, of course, is most clear in the case of schools, where the public has been made aware that there are many children with serious problems with whom teachers are relatively ineffective. That situation is by no means new; what is new is the public's recognition that the situation is indeed so serious that it should no longer be tolerated. That recognition has brought in its wake myriad proposals for change, *none* of which, unfortunately, speaks directly to the clinical nature of teaching; that is, to the number of times during a day that a teacher must deal with troubled children and parents. They are proposals imprisoned in the imagery of a teacher standing before a class of (usually) seated children: informing, instructing, stimulating, correcting, disciplining, and so on. It is imagery as unrealistic as it is prepotent. We are, as I indicated in the previous chapter, beginning to recognize that many lawyers are in clinical roles about which they feel both ambivalent and unprepared, but that knowledge has hardly seeped into the public's awareness, although it has into that of researchers. Unlike medicine and teaching, where some practitioners have articulated concern about the inadequacies of the preparation for the clinical role, in the field of law there have been very few who have posed or discussed the problem.

There are several reasons for emphasizing the commonalities in clinical functions among these different fields. First, the perception of commonalities is an instance of how inevitably imprisoned we have been in our culture: its symbols, the differentiations we are taught and accept, and the social definitions of roles that serve as a compass for directing individual and group actions. The perception of commonalities shocks us, so to speak, in that we are made aware that we have been confusing surface difference with underlying similarities—phenotype with genotype. Second, the perception of commonalities in fields heretofore regarded as having literally quite different cores raises the possibility that these fields have something to learn from each other, especially if one or more of them is viewed as more highly developed in regard to what they have in common. There is, of course, the possibility that, in regard to this common core, none of them has squarely or effectively confronted the issues this common core poses. This is the possibility I have discussed in this book in regard to what constitutes caring and compassionate actions in those engaged in the clinical endeavor. Third, because prevention of problems is incomparably superior to efforts at repair, the perception of commonalities increases the opportunities to gain new insights about how the clinical and preventive orientations can be integrated. As I have emphasized in previous chapters, to the extent that a clinician focuses on helping *an* individual, the opportunities for primary, secondary, and tertiary prevention have been drastically narrowed. The very fact that we tend to view the labels *clinical* and *prevention* as polarities has been a mammoth obstacle to clarity, rooted as that obstacle is in our educational and training institutions, where prevention is here and the clinical endeavor is there and never shall the twain meet, conceptually and practically.

Finally, the perception of commonalities provides a basis for judging whether explanations of deficiencies in the clinical endeavor—such as those proffered to explain the lack of caring and compassionate behavior among teachers and physicians—have merit. If the same deficiencies exist in fields that are strikingly different from each other on the surface but that nevertheless have an important common core, then an explanation of deficiencies in common core in one field should, to some degree at least, have explanatory relevance for those same deficiencies in other fields. More concretely, how should we view past and present explanations of and remedies for the relative lack of caring and compassionate behavior among physicians? What if those explanations indict factors and contexts minimally or not at all present in other clinical fields where the same deficiencies exist?

It is conceivable, of course, that the same deficiencies can arise under very different circumstances, but it is possible—indeed, likely—that, despite these different circumstances, the explanation of these deficiencies has generality rather than particularity or uniqueness. In light of the previous chapters, it will come as no surprise to the reader that I believe that these deficiencies are, to a very important extent, independent of the differences in contexts among the fields comprising the clinical endeavor. *Differences in contexts are differences that make a difference but are by no means the whole story.* And if they are by no means the whole story, then remedies that call for changes in context (for example, changing the curriculum, altering the distribution of power) cannot be expected to have a powerful effect. Modifying what exists is one thing: recognizing what has been absent but is crucially important is quite another thing. If it is understandable that we tend to change only what we think we know how to change, it should be no less understandable that that with which we are familiar and comfortable often prevents us from asking: What are we not thinking about that we should be thinking about but that we would not know how to think about or act in regard to, or, if we did, that would mean that we would be traveling a very lonely road?

Because issues surrounding caring and compassion in the clinical endeavor have been most recognized and discussed in medicine, we will use that congery of fields as a basis for making comparative judgments of explanations of why those issues have arisen. Let us start with Flexner's assumption that a liberal arts education is the best insurance for inculcating in physicians a caring and compassionate understanding of self, troubled individuals, and their families; that is, that it provides an understanding of people, their works, and their histories that makes "insight and sympathy" possible and likely. Current critics do not question Flexner's assumptions. On the contrary, they relate uncaring and uncompassionate behavior among physicians to the fact that since Flexner's time the undergraduate education of physicians has contained less and less of the liberal arts. The goal, it is said, should be to restore the liberal arts as a prerequisite for a career in medicine. How relevant is this explanation in the case of those who seek careers in those parts of law and psychology that are clinical in nature?

However one defines a liberal arts education, it is safe to assume that, compared to physicians, those entering psychology and law have sampled more widely in the liberal arts, with those entering law school probably sampling most widely. Are lawyers and psychologists in their clinical roles more caring and compassionate than physicians? The answer is that we do not know. I am talking here not about attitudes and values but about observable behavior in the clinical situation. I have had over forty years of experience in clinical psychology. My experience with medical students and physicians is less but still considerable, and I have had less but by no means minuscule experience with lawyers. The one conclusion that I feel most secure in stating is that, at best, the correlation between caring and compassionate behavior, on the one hand, and degree of exposure to the liberal arts, on the other hand, is positive but small. And there are times when I have concluded that the correlation is zero. And what about teachers? They are a very instructive group, because, up until World War II, many teachers (especially in elementary schools) received their post–high school education either in two-year "normal schools" or in colleges devoted exclusively to training teachers. One of the major reasons these schools disappeared was the criticism that teachers lacking a liberal arts education simply did not have the basis for productive teaching; that is, they were technicians, hardly to be considered professionals. In recent years, the criticism has taken the form of the recommendation that professional training in education should begin only after a four-year liberal arts education. In any event, despite increased exposure to the liberal arts, there is no evidence whatsoever that the quality of teaching has discernibly improved. Indeed, teachers have been subject to the criticism that, as a group, they, like physicians, are not as caring and compassionate as they should be.

I am, of course, in no way derogating a liberal arts education. I am calling into question the assumption that a liberal arts education instills in students that kind of knowledge and attitude that produces understanding leading to caring and compassionate behavior. Put in another way, why should the acquisition of fact, abstractions, and generalizations, devoid of any integration with or application to concrete situations that test understanding, be expected to influence behavior in desired ways? One could argue that it could or should have such an influence, and I would so argue, but that is quite different from saying that it does. It is more than an act of faith on my part to believe that a liberal arts education can and does have many benefits over the course of one's life, but it is far from self-evident that among these benefits are its effects on how one understands, responds to, and "treats" other people.

My conclusion is vulnerable to the criticism that I am asking too much of a college liberal arts education. The goal is not to produce "finished products" but rather to broaden horizons, to inculcate humanistic values, and to provide a basis for deciding on a career that will allow one to lead a satisfying personal, intellectual, and ethical existence. The liberal arts provide one with building blocks, so to speak, from which one's personal house can begin to be built, and that building takes place after college; for example, in some graduate field or professional school. Education in the liberal arts is only a beginning, a kind of capital that one has acquired for later investment. For my purposes here, I accept that criticism, but I have to point out that it concedes the argument that, by itself, a liberal arts education should not be expected to produce caring and compassionate people—in Flexner's terms, people with "requisite insight and sympathy." And such an unrealistic expectation gives added force to a second explanation of the frequency of uncaring and uncompassionate actions, to which we now turn.

The second explanation, again in relation to medical education, has several parts, but they can all be subsumed under the following statement: Medical schools effectively cure students of the tendency to give overt expression to caring and compassionate feelings. Undue competitiveness, acquisition of facts that strain memory, being made to feel ignorant and incompetent, being socialized to worship at the shrines of science and technology, being influenced by mentors who are verbally caring and compassionate but in action are otherwise, being warned against getting "overinvolved" with patients—these are some of the features of the medical school experience that critics point to in explaining the frequency with which physicians are uncaring and uncompassionate. When we look at law schools, we encounter many of the same features, despite the obvious cultural-educational-structural differences between law and medical schools. The message, directly and indirectly articulated, is that the law has a tradition and logic that are and should be independent of subjective feelings about what is right and wrong, fair and unfair. One of the major problems of the law student is to accommodate to a way of logical thinking, to a way of identifying principles and precedent, that is divorced from the student's sense of interpersonal and social justice and morality. The law has a logic that has little to do with psychology. I must make mention here of a recent study by Marsh (1985) concerned in part with the perceptions of medical and law students of their educational experience. She interviewed first- and fourth-year medical students and first- and third-year law students. One of the questions she asked specifically concerned how they perceived the influence of their professional education on their sense of caring and compassion. Here is her summary of what these students said:

> The question about caring and compassion seemed, for many subjects, to be a key to unlocking their very pressing concerns about how they were being changed by their training, and about why their objections to some of those changes were not recognized by those in power of the profession. Many subjects, who had been somewhat constricted in their responses up to that point, suddenly breathed a sigh of relief at the question, as if it had struck an important chord.
>
> The question seemed to invite the subjects to complain about their training and their fields. Responses would typically begin with the subject's listing all the complaints about the profession, which interfere with compassion. At some point, the tone would shift from one of complaining, to one of explaining why it was so difficult for compassion to exist in that climate. For some subjects, this tone would traverse the fine line into justifying why compassion was really counter-productive to the main tenets of the profession. The vacillation, from complaining, to explaining, to justifying, and back again, was frequent for some subjects, perhaps dependent on the degree of conflict the subjects felt in reconciling their own values to the values of their profession. It often sounded as if the subjects were trying to convince themselves of the justice of their new ideas. When that conviction didn't hold, they'd slip back again to a different intonation.
>
> The law students expressed a sense of guilt, stemming from two factors. The first was guilt over the fact that they would be making money in their careers, frequently by joining large corporate firms, as opposed to doing something that they could see

as more socially useful. In addition to the monetary question, however, they expressed guilt over an exquisite awareness that they were being presented with a version of the law that made personal feelings irrelevant. In order to adopt the professional code of legal ethics, they realized that they would have to set aside their own set of moral values.

This message is the same one that was communicated to medical students, which stipulated that the expression of feelings was at odds with the attempt to maintain a professional demeanor. Medical students were taught to strip away their natural feelings toward the patients as human beings, and to regard their patients as mere biological entities.

The picture in colleges of education is quite different. In contrast to students in medical and law schools, the teacher in training is told in myriad ways the importance of understanding, caring, and compassion. If anything, the message to the student is that the teacher has to be a psychological diagnostician who uses his or her perceptions and feelings to understand and to adapt to the differences among students. The teacher should be caring and compassionate, prepared to give overt expression to such feelings in ways that are helpful to a child within the constraints of the characteristics of that particular class. The maxim "you teach children, not subject matter" underlines the interpersonal emphasis without which teaching is an arid affair and the classroom a bore.

If the message to the prospective teacher is so different from that communicated to law and medical students, why are teachers so frequently seen as uncaring and uncompassionate? There are many reasons, but, for my present purposes, I shall discuss only those that speak to what the prospective teacher experiences (or does not) in the course of training. The first inheres in being "told": teachers are "told" the message, they "hear" it, they "accept" it, but it is on a general level so divorced from concrete example or setting as to justify labeling the message as a cliché. If such a label is pejorative, it is not because clichés lack substantive validity (they do not), but rather because they give no direction to action that would appropriately reflect its substance. I have never heard an educator disagree with the cliché that "you teach children, not subject matter." What does that mean for a teacher in a classroom? By what criteria does a teacher know that he or she is acting consistently with the intent of a cliché? The fact is that what teachers learn about caring and compassion, about understanding the needs of a child, they almost always learn in courses unrelated to a live classroom or any other setting in which children are found. But does not the prospective teacher have to fulfill the requirement of practice teaching?

That question brings us to the second reason: although the period of practice teaching varies from program to program, it rarely exceeds two or three months. When you realize how much we expect teachers to know and to be able to do—to productively wed complicated theory to complicated practice—the usual duration of practice teaching is both inexplicable and inexcusable. (When John Dewey said that schoolteachers should be paid as much as college teachers, it was testimony to the respect he had for what a schoolteacher needed to know, understand, and be able to do.) Duration aside, the period of practice teaching is one in which the technical-methodological features of teaching receive the most attention. I am not suggesting that these features are unimportant, but when they receive far more attention than the development of the teacher as psychological observer, diagnostician, and clinician, it should not occasion surprise that teachers so frequently are viewed as insensitive applied psychologists unable to recognize and help troubled children. So, despite the fact that the messages teachers receive in their preparatory years are discernibly different from those that law and medical students hear, the end result is similar. And I say similar and not identical, because, in my experience, more than medical and law students, teachers as a group want and try to be understanding, caring, and compassionate but are puzzled and disappointed with the consequences their actions in such a stance lead them to take. Teachers are among the most articulate critics of the inadequacy and even irrelevancy of their preparation for life in a classroom and school.

When we turn to psychiatry and clinical psychology, the picture changes somewhat, in emphasis, at least. More so than in any of the other fields I have discussed, the trainee is exposed to and is expected to absorb a particular theoretical view of human behavior. Theories abound in these fields; they are taken very seriously on the level of lecture, discussion, and research; and they are sources of controversy and polarization. Each training program tends to be wedded to a particular theoretical orientation; usually one other orientation is represented, but to a subordinate degree. The message to the student is that theory ("this" theory) is important, indeed absolutely necessary, for productive research and effective clinical action. I have no quarrel with that except that it is a message correlated with another message, more subtle and usually unverbalized (except in departmental meetings): the trainee who has a flair for theory and research is better or more worthy or more respected than the trainee who does not. The trainee who is perceived to be a good clinician but weak or uninterested in theory and research is not derogated, of course, but neither is he or she rated high on the academic scale of ultimate worthiness. Trainees have no difficulty hearing the message and perceiving its consequences. And one of those consequences is that, when engaged in research, the trainee is supervised by a member of the full-time faculty, while clinical work is supervised (far more often than not) by a practitioner in the community or an advanced trainee. It sounds strange, and I realize that it is not consciously intended, that programs whose goal it is to train clinicians tend to devalue those who will spend their lives in the clinical endeavor. And if they do not devalue them, they are certainly ambivalent in their feelings toward them.

The trainee is very much aware that he or she is being indoctrinated in regard to a theory and socialized into the role of psychological clinician. And the trainee early on experiences an internal conflict in regard to the clinical role, between what he or she spontaneously feels about and wants to express to a client and the requirement of objectivity without which one can be led into harmful actions. To be objective, as in conducting research, means not that one is without strong feeling but rather that such feeling has to be controlled so that it does not get injected into and distort the phenomena one is studying. The analyst behind the couch is the clinical counterpart of the objective scientist. But even where the psychoanalytical orientation is not the dominant one, the trainee is not left in doubt about the need for objectivity; that is, to make sure that the boundaries between client and patient are not blurred. The tendency of the trainee to want to give expression to feeling (to soothe, sympathize with, pass judgment, take sides) is seen as "normal" but potentially very dangerous; that is, as antitherapeutic overinvolvement.

On the surface, trainees accept the need for objectivity—it does have the ring of science, and its importance can be illustrated with examples of the baleful consequences of "emotional overinvolvement"—but internally there is a struggle, as one of my students put it, "between what your heart says you should say and do and what theory and your supervisor say you should say and do." Many trainees give up the struggle, but there are some who continue to feel that in striving to maintain the stance of objectivity they are robbing themselves and their clients of something of therapeutic value. The trainee's struggle, which supervisors gloss over as a normal developmental phase that trainees grow out of, points to an omission in psychological-psychiatric theories. Those theories never concern themselves with caring and compassion. What does it mean to be caring and compassionate? When do caring and compassion arise as feelings? What inhibits or facilitates their expression? Why do people differ so widely in having such feelings and in the ways they express them? It is, of course, implicit in all of these theories that these feelings are crucial in human development, but the reader would be surprised how little attention is given to their phenomenology and consequences (positive and negative). Credit can be given to Freud for recognizing that, on the level of clinical action, the spontaneous feelings that the clinical interaction engenders in the therapist are very important. But Freud deserves the criticism that, in emphasizing the importance of objectivity, indeed impersonality, he was instilling in the therapist feelings and actions of potential therapeutic value. Freud made a virtue of objectivity, although, when you read about his relationships with patients, you find that he was far from the objective, neutral, passive observer and responder.

A noted psychologist, Kurt Lewin, once said that there is nothing more practical than a good theory; that is, a good theory serves as a map of and a compass for traversing the psychological terrain. But how well does extant theory map the terrain? In 1935, John Dollard—a sociologist, anthropologist, psychoanalyst, and psychologist—pointed out in a truly seminal book (Dollard, 1935) that psychological-psychiatric theories were egregiously incomplete and misleading, because they were so inadequate in conceptualizing human behavior in its cultural contexts. What was at stake was not only how one *interpreted* psychological phenomena and saw them in their developmental aspects but how those interpretations influenced the clinician's actions. When Dollard wrote that book, the psychological clinician worked mostly with white, middle-class, suburban individuals. Today, as I indicated in an earlier chapter, the clinician is confronted with client groups far more diverse in cultural background, ethnicity, and race. Unfortunately, Dollard's 1935 critique is as cogent today as it was then in that neither the theories to which trainees are exposed nor the supervision they receive adequately prepare them for understanding individuals differing markedly from them in background. And that inadequacy on the part of the trainee and supervisor impoverishes their understanding and makes caring and compassionate actions a sometime thing. Furthermore, when one examines training programs, one is struck by the restricted range in cultural background of the clients that trainees see. Despite the recognition psychiatry and clinical psychology pay to the importance of cultural, racial, ethnic, and gender factors, the modal curriculum is blatantly deficient in exposing the trainee, both in theory and in practice, to the implications of those factors for the clinical endeavor. In this respect, these two fields share this deficiency with education.

The fields of medicine, law, education, and psychology are very different kinds of places in the university, but, on the level of rhetoric, they differ not at all in the respect they pay to the importance of instilling in their students sensitivity to the needs and feelings of those they seek to help. On the level of practice, however, the rhetoric is undercut, or underemphasized, or simply contradicted. Precisely because this occurs in fields differing so obviously in tradition, history, structure, and curriculum, one has to go beyond these differences for explanation. Such an explanation is far beyond the scope of this book, but one part of such an explanation will be taken up in the next chapter.

It has been argued that, although training centers are part of the problem, the nature of the "real world" into which students are catapulted when they have finished their training plays no less of a role, perhaps a far greater one, in diluting the sense of caring and compassion. The argument identifies two factors: the inexorable dynamics of earning a livelihood and the consequences of the increasing tendency for clinicians to work in or to be related to large, bureaucratic organizations. In regard to earning a living, it is pointed out that many students finish their training heavily in debt, they have start-up expenses, and they already are at an age when they feel they must make up for "lost time." Time—as something to be made up and something to be filled in by as many income-producing activities as possible—becomes the crucial determinant; and, of course, one of its consequences is that the needs of clients are subtly and sometimes consciously defined in terms of the clinician's perception of time constraints. This is particularly the case when the clinician is "successful": he or she has many clients making myriad demands on the clinician's time. The clinician becomes a rationer of time, and that obviously sets drastic limits on the degree to which the ever-present client need for caring and compassion can be met. The display of caring and compassion cannot be done by formula, it is not synonymous with verbal platitudes, and its requirements cannot be governed by clock time. And, let us not forget, the striving for understanding that precedes and is essential for caring and compassionate actions also requires time. In short, when it is said that the economics of clinical practice tend to interfere with caring and compassionate actions, reference is being made to time as a limited and precious resource that must be husbanded and rationed. But it also refers to and accepts the fact that the clinician, like any enterprising business person, seeks to maximize income. And, as with the business person, the level of income deemed both necessary and desirable reflects a conception of what is required for "the good life."

The economic argument is strange in several ways, and by *strange,* I refer to what the argument implies and what it leaves out. For one thing, the argument implies and sometimes comes close to saying that the clinician is *in business,* that, like it or not, the clinician's outlook and actions are mightily determined by time and money. Put in a more stark way: it is now a fiction to say that the clinician's behavior is solely determined by the needs of clients. This is not to say that the needs of clients are not in the picture—that would be a grossly unfair exaggeration—but rather that we are in a time when the clinical interaction is increasingly being influenced by considerations unrelated to the needs of clients but very much related to the way clinicians define their own needs.

Clinicians in the health fields can talk long and loud about the constraints put upon them by public policies, legislation, court decisions, and, of course, the seemingly endless amount of rulings and paper work that comes with one or another type of private and public health insurance. In no small measure, their resentment stems from the inroads these factors make on their time, not only in terms of filling out forms but in keeping up with changes in rules governing payment and having to take the time to explain these changes to office staff and clients and not infrequently having to take time to battle insurance companies about fee schedules. Although these angry clinicians leave no doubt in one's mind about how these irritations and constraints interfere with their sense of autonomy, they have never said that the interference spills over into their relations with clients. It is as if, when they are closeted with their clients, the outside world that is in both the clinician and client is stilled and inoperative. It is a view that confuses hope with reality, or intention with practice. The fact is that at least on a dozen occasions I had the opportunity to talk individually to clinicians of varying types (some in private practice, some in agencies and hospitals, and some not in practice but in top administrative positions), to whom I said that it was inconceivable to me that clinicians could assert that their relations with clients were not affected by the purely businesslike demands on conducting a practice *and* maintaining a good income. All but one agreed completely with me, although only four of them would say that there were times when their reactions to clients had been adversely affected, if only minimally. But all of them said they knew clinicians for whom the label *business person* was both appropriate and pejorative, and that there was every reason to believe that their numbers were on the increase. I should also note that four of these clinicians were sixty years of age or more. They had become clinicians long before private health insurance became widespread, governmental health programs (Medicare, Medicaid, Supplemental Social Security programs, and so on) had been instituted, and the meteoric increase in the size and cast of health care was envisioned. I know how easy it is to look back on "the good old days" when presumably virtue reigned, people were "called" to the clinical endeavor, and self and family sacrifice was necessary (indeed, natural) and understood as the price to be paid for being able to do good for sick and troubled people. As one of these senior (citizen) clinicians said:

> We worked like dogs in medical school and in the internship, but we *expected* to, and if we bitched and griped, we also loved almost every goddamned minute of it. We were learning, we were doing, we depended on each other, we were part of a real fraternity. And when we went into practice, we expected to be called to someone's home in the middle of the night and on Sunday. We wished they didn't call, but we didn't have an unlisted number, or an answering service that said we could not be reached, and we didn't view it as unwar-

ranted intrusion into our privacy if we got calls at home. One thing we were not: businessmen. We took account of what a patient could afford, not what his nonexistent policy could pay for. We had no gravy trains like Medicare or policies that some of the corporations and the federal government arrange for their employees that are so tempting to a physician that wants to make an easy buck. The physician going into practice today quickly becomes a businessman. He already knows about health insurance, the ins and outs of third-party payments, and the importance of an accountant to tell you how to beat the tax laws. Patients are persons, but they are also fees. When you go to a physician for the first time, what is the first question you are asked by his receptionist? Do you have insurance? If not, how will you pay? I entered the game before all of these so-called great and wonderful changes took place. I feel like an outsider. I also feel very, very old! And I hate to admit it, but there are days when I want to say to some of my complaining patients: "How about listening to some of my complaints? How about holding my hand? Who will be my confessor?" And when I hear younger physicians complain about being overworked, and when I see them become part of a group in order to reduce the time they have to spend with patients, and when their stationery has after their name P.C. for professional corporation, and when some of them have *never,* but *never,* been in a patient's home and can see no reason why they ever should, and some of them talk as if God created patients to elevate and caress their egos—I must admit that I get angry, feel alone, and yet feel good about myself.

I am not about to assert that the good old days were as good as this physician suggested. I should point out that there is a rather large literature by physicians (or members of their family) that in all respects confirms the contrast the physician whose fifteen-minute outburst I paraphrased tried to describe. Setting aside how good the good old days were, no one denies that economic factors—as perceived by the clinician, the client, or the larger society—have affected to an undetermined extent the clinician-client relationship, especially in regard to the clinician's display of caring and compassionate behavior. The clinical endeavor is in the process of becoming a business endeavor, and what I find strange is that the implications of that process have barely been studied. For example, I know of no study that has sought to determine how and to what extent (if any) third-party payments have altered the nature, duration, and quality of clinician-client interactions. After all, payment through third parties represents a dramatic economic alteration in the basis of clinician-client contact, and what permits us to assume that it has not been accompanied by alterations in the interpersonal aspects of the contact, of which issues surrounding caring and compassion may be but one aspect? I find it very strange in light of the billions of dollars that have been poured in the post–World War II period into the research endeavor in the health fields, and in light of the concerns expressed during this same period about the absence or weakening of caring and compassion among health professionals, that those concerns have for all practical purposes gone unresearched. It is a strange omission, although it is by no means strange that fields of professional practice are wary of self-scrutiny. But the issues go far beyond any one field in that they suggest that we are paying too high a price for what we have been led to believe is undiluted progress. It is a societal or public-policy issue in that it concerns the means and ends that characterize vitally significant human relationships.

The economic-time explanation is strange in still another way, because it fails to note that the identical explanation is advanced to explain some of the inadequacies in professional training; for example, the duration of training programs, time constraints on the curriculum and faculty. Indeed, nowhere more than in the years of training do the pressures and preciousness of time suffuse the phenomenology of everyone and get used to justify an admittedly distorted integration of means and ends. In this respect, what the clinician experiences after finishing training is a continuation of an attitude, of a way of structuring professional life, that was absorbed before entering practice. On finishing training, the clinician is catapulted into a "real world," but it is one that in regard to the time-economic argument he or she has encountered before.

The second major explanation for the weakening of caring and compassionate actions points to the increasing tendency for clinicians to work full time in large, bureaucratic organizations—large hospitals, larger medical centers, health maintenance organizations, state or federal facilities, and profit-making corporations that in recent years have become a significant factor in the "health industry" (for example, Starr, 1982; Wahl, 1984). It is an explanation that conjures up the familiar imagery of an organization differentiated and complicated in structure, the parts of which have boundaries that are far from permeable, governed by policies and rules made and distributed in a top-down fashion, all of this rationalized in terms of a more efficient and effective provision of clinical services, and all of this adversely affecting not only the autonomy of the clinician but the quality of the clinical interaction. If this imagery is one with which increasing numbers of clinicians are becoming familiar, it has long been familiar to educators, especially those in our urban school systems. In fact, some critics of education have asserted that teachers are not professionals, because they are not able to determine or control the conditions in which they render services—what they teach, when they teach, and even how they teach are determined and controlled by others. These critics indict teachers, teachers indict "the system," the system in turn indicts teachers, and commission after commission bemoans the quality of life in schools and the fate of students. In the current debate about how to improve our schools, much is made of attracting a better quality of person to teaching, as if the performance of teachers is independent of the bureaucratic features of the school system. I said earlier that, in my experience, teachers, more than physicians and lawyers, want and try to be compassionate in their efforts to help children. They recognize the inadequacies of their preparation for the clinical endeavor, but they also have no difficulty illustrating how the system in which they work can prevent them from being helpful, or even trying to be helpful, and cause them to give up trying. *Burnout* has become a fashionable term in educational circles and is used both to explain and to excuse the uncaring and uncompassionate stance. To the extent that the tendency for health professionals to work in organizations continues, they will confront all of the dilemmas attendant to being in Max Weber's "iron cage." But, I must emphasize, those dilemmas cannot be explained simply by what I call organizational craziness. Unfortunately, those poignant dilemmas are confronted and then put on the back burner, so to speak, during the years of training. In effect, clinicians are being socialized, unwittingly, of course, to make them adaptable to the role of the organization clinician.

In 1975, a physician, Charles Harris, wrote a personal memoir, *One Man's Medicine* (Harris, 1975). Harris came to medicine well before the health fields took on the features of large industry. The following is from the prologue to his book:

> As we struggle to attain a higher plane of social organization, the physician becomes increasingly subordinate to organizations, governments, institutions, and men of neither license nor tradition in medicine, who have vaulted into positions of power in the newly created health syndicate: businessmen, lawyers, accountants, car salesmen, bankers and the new breed, the hospital administrator; paper doctors who treat paper. They see to the health of the by-laws, procedure manuals, bills, accounts, debits and insurance forms, beguiled by the delusion that if the records are neat and orderly, institutional care of the patients is neat and orderly.
>
> The doctor, as their hireling, is forced to use the tools and services they provide, which may not be the best available; urged to consider the commu-

nity as a whole when treating his patient; coerced
into violating the confidentiality of the doctor-
patient relationship by monitoring the utilization
of hospital beds by his colleagues.

Nurses resent being "handmaidens" to the
doctor, and strive to become an independent profession.

There is a hue and cry for doctors to divest
themselves of the elite position they have held so
long in medicine. Who, then, should be the elite?

Clearly the precious bond that exists between a patient and his doctor is being riven by
unqualified intruders with unlimited power. The
physician, in his spiritual and serving role, may be
the commodity that is squandered in this struggle.

The medical profession is increasingly in
bondage. Like the point of an inverted pyramid it
is being pressed deeper into the ground by the
weight of an enlarging, expensive bureaucracy. If
the profession of medicine is shattered by this burden, would it be asking too much for Aesculapius
to be reborn? [pp. ix–x].

What Harris said in print is what many physicians of his genera-
tion have told me in private. One does not have to agree with
everything Harris says, but one cannot deny that the transformations against which he so eloquently rails raise the question:
The clinician is whose agent? As soon as the clinician becomes
part of the organization, he or she becomes an agent of that
organization, and it is indulging wishful thinking to believe that
Harris's "precious bond" between clinician and client will not
be affected. As I have said before, caring and compassion are
not platonic essences people carry around inside of them; they
are terms intended to describe qualities of the transactions between people. And when in those transactions the clinician has
divided loyalties—worse yet, when the dissonance created by
divided loyalties has succumbed to the pressure to conform—
caring and compassion will be neither a frequent nor a distinc-

tive feature of the clinical interaction. At the least, let us recognize that being caring and compassionate has been made more problematic.

What is distinctive about the current scene is the rate at which clinicians are employed in bureaucratic settings. The fact is that clinicians have long been employed in these settings: mental hospitals, training schools for the mentally retarded, reformatories, prisons, VA hospitals. These settings have long and complicated histories, but one feature they have always shared—beginning with Dorothea Dix's descriptions in 1848—is the absence of caring and compassionate ambience. To my knowledge, no one has ever brought together in a book the scandalous conditions that countless exposés have described in these settings over the past century and a half. It is probably not an exaggeration that, in the post–World War II era, not a month has gone by without at least one such exposé and/or one such setting being put under the jurisdiction of a state or federal court. And if one includes nursing homes, the number would be higher. These conditions, of course, cannot be laid at the doorstep of clinicians, but that does not negate the fact that clinicians were part of and tolerated inhumane treatments and conditions. And that is the point: these clinicians were mired in a complicated setting and saw themselves powerless to act caringly and compassionately in their clinical roles.

I had the enlightening experience of beginning my professional career in 1942 in a spanking-new state institution for the mentally retarded where, for the first two years, it would be correct to say that the institution existed for its patients. But after that, slowly and subtly, it would be no less correct to say that the needs of the residents became secondary to intrainstitutional needs created by growth, departmental rivalry, professional-imperialistic battles, and state rules and regulations. Whose agent I was became a pressing, daily moral problem. I know what it is to have divided loyalties, to want to give up the fight, to rationalize away the internalized conflict. Matters were not helped any by the knowledge that the professional fields and organizations to which I and other types of clinicians belonged viewed us as outside the professional mainstream, a view that rendered these clinical fields insensitive to issues that later would haunt them when mainstream health settings would begin to increase in size and employ large numbers of clinicians on a full-time basis. We are a society that tends to confuse growth with progress. Nowhere is this more true than in the clinical professions, where exponential growth was enthusiastically embraced as a sign that the quality and quantity of clinical services would follow as a matter of course. If this embrace is being subjected to a second look, if only by a minority of clinical educators, it is, unfortunately, not based on knowledge derived from the long history of these clinical fields in complex organizations. If they were aware of this history, their level of concern would noticeably increase, and their thinking and recommendations might become appropriately more radical.

In light of the tendency for clinicians to be employed in ever-growing, complex organizations, this question arises: In what ways and to what extent do training centers in our universities alert their students to the dynamics of and the issues surrounding the "whose agent am I" question? That question can be put in another way: What do these students learn about working in complex bureaucratic organizations where divided loyalties is a predictable problem that will have an impact on their ability to act caringly and compassionately? I prefer the second form of the question, because it diverts attention to a dramatic alteration in where clinicians are and will be increasingly working. Why, someone could argue, do students have to be exposed to this inasmuch as the centers that train them are (or are part of) large, complicated settings with which they are familiar? Or, someone else could argue, are not students frequently in the position where they are in conflict between what they would like to do to help a patient and what their supervisor or the rules and regulations of the setting require them to do?

To the first question, one has to note that the fact that the student receives training in this type of setting is no warrant for assuming that the student understands and has validly conceptualized the setting so as to permit transfer of that understanding to the settings in which he or she may be later employed. In my experience, at least, what students on their own learn about these training centers they regard as unique to these centers; that is, they are settings whose features they will not encounter again. To the second question (whose agent am I?), the answer is that there is a world of difference between experiencing the problem in the role of student and in the role of full-fledged clinician who does not have a supervisor to whom one is accountable for decisions in regard to every client. Yes, the student experiences the agency issue, but only infrequently as a truly moral issue. The student is primarily the supervisor's agent, not the client's; that is understood from the very beginning.

In any event, I do not pretend to have done an exhaustive survey of clinical curricula or to have interviewed scores of students and their mentors, but I have done enough to feel secure in concluding that the issues surrounding "whose agent am I?" receive short shrift or no attention at all. Training centers pay obeisance to ethical and moral issues in clinical work; for example, a few lectures, an elective course, a special lecture series, or a special symposium to address an issue (Baby Jane Doe, recombinant DNA, test-tube fertilization, terminating life of someone with "dead brain") that has gripped public interest and requires a public policy. But they are not exposed to the nature of organizations and how their dynamics will affect clinical practice in general and caring and compassionate actions in particular. And this failure is due not only to a lack of understanding of transformations in the society that have long been picking up a head of steam but also to the absence of a research focus on the behavior of clinicians. We know a good deal about what clinicians say about what and how they do, and we know how many recipients of clinicians' behavior have said they reacted, varying from undiluted praise to vitriolic anger. But a systematic focus on what actually goes on has yet to emerge.

The concerns I have expressed in these pages have in the past year been articulated within medicine; for example, by President Bok (1984) of Harvard University, the Association of Medical Colleges (1984), and some deans of medical schools. If there is agreement on anything in regard to recommendations, it is that means must be found that would make it possible for a person to withstand the pressures in the undergraduate years to avoid a truly broad liberal arts education. It is recognized, however, that such means cannot be counted on to withstand the ambience of medical schools, which apparently few if any knowledgeable people regard as interpersonally healthy in the sense that it is conducive to assimilating caring and compassionate attitudes and actions. Introducing new courses into the curriculum and trying out a new curriculum with a small part of the entering class and with selected members of the medical faculty have been recommended and will be implemented. One can expect that these efforts, particularly those in prestigious medical schools, will be imitated elsewhere.

At the same time that I am encouraged by the clarity of the articulated concerns, and respectful of the new efforts precisely because of their purposes, there are several reasons why I am not optimistic that the goals of these efforts will be achieved, even in small part. For one thing, the history of curriculum reform in any field does not warrant optimism about the impact of curriculum on attitudes and behaviors. Insofar as introducing a "humanistic" emphasis in medical education is concerned, curriculum reform in the past has been a failure. In the field of education—notably in the sixties in regard to the new math, new biology, and new social studies—the same conclusion is warranted, as I have discussed elsewhere (Sarason, 1982). Substituting one curriculum for another is no great feat, done as it usually is by fiat by those with power. There is a difference between exercising power and exercising wisdom, and the difference resides in how well one understands the different vested interests that will be confronted by the change, the difference between formal and informal power, the strength of institutional traditions, and the relationship of these considerations to the determination of a realistic time perspective. Far from being a narrow technical process, curriculum reform is a test of the relation between complicated theory and practice, and the history of curriculum reform is replete with instances where that relation was superficially recognized, when it was recognized at all. This means not that curriculum reform has failed in any

total sense (although that appears to be the case in recent decades in medical education) but rather that the major purposes
of the reforms were hardly achieved. For example, the introduction of the new math in the late fifties and sixties was heralded
as a way to make the learning of math "enjoyable." Leaving
aside whatever positive effects the new math may have had, the
fact remains that the goal of making the new math an enjoyable
experience for student *and* teacher remains an unachieved goal.
And again I must make reference to Flexner. His effort at reform of the medical curriculum in 1910 was successful in that it
wedded medicine and science, but in regard to his goal of training physicians who were caring and compassionate—whose regard for people would be no less than their regard for the truths
of science—his effort turned out to be counterproductive.

The outcomes of curriculum reform have to be evaluated
in terms of stated goals. Today, in medicine, law, psychology,
and education, the goal that is coming into center stage is implicit in the question: What kind of person do we want the clinician to be, and how do we help such a person become that?
That question is quite different from asking what we want a
clinician to know and to be able to do in a technical sense. We
want a clinician to know his or her craft, and we have a pretty
good idea (and a lot of experience) about what technical competence in a craft consists of. But precisely because clinicians
deal with events and problems fateful in the lives of their clients, we want clinicians to exercise their craft in as caring and
compassionate a way as possible. We do not want the clinician
to forget that achieving technical goals is not an end that should
ever be judged independent of the interpersonal sensitivity that
should precede and accompany technical achievement. The surgeon who is a masterful craftsperson, the teacher who has mas-
tered subject matter and pedagogical technique, the lawyer
thoroughly sophisticated about divorce law, the mental health
clinician deeply knowledgeable about the tactics of influence
and persuasion—in all of these instances, we hope for more than
technical knowledge and skill; we hope for understanding, caring, and compassion and that sense that our symptoms and problems are not treated in isolation from what we are and need,

from what we are as persons. (I am not my appendix, I am not my reading problem, I am not my phobia, I am not my divorce!)

What kind of a person do we want a clinician to be? It is egregiously superficial to answer that question in terms of narrow, technical outcomes. And when that kind of answer is rather routinely given to excuse the absence of caring and compassionate behavior, we can be secure in concluding that a similar excuse will be given to explain their absence in many other areas of human relationships. What kind of a person do we want a clinician to be? How shall we live with each other? Some people dismiss these questions as (pejoratively) philosophical, reflecting the concerns of people who are at best impractical and at worst adolescently utopian. The fact is that these are the questions that are coming to concern the professional community, because, inexorably, albeit inchoately, they have come to sense that something is very wrong somewhere, that the "precious bond" between clinician and client has begun to be severered, with disquieting effects on client and clinician alike. The number of clinicians who feel this way is not small, although the number who articulate and write about it is small. But there are few clinicians who are not aware that the abstraction that we call the general public has in recent decades become very critical of those in the clinical endeavor. And at the top of the list of criticisms is that too many clinicians are not very caring and compassionate people, however technically competent they may be. Ironically, there is one factor that may well keep this criticism from militantly erupting: people no longer expect to be treated caringly and compassionately. Just as the clinician in a large organization tends to succumb to organizational pressures, so does the experience of clients with clinicians lead them to lower expectations.

In current discussions about reform in the clinical professions, little or no attention has been given to how candidates are selected. Dissatisfaction is voiced about the undue weight given to scores on admission tests or to piling up of the kind of course directly related to the chosen clinical field. This criticism indicts these criteria because they are "successful": they predict well who will finish their graduate work, but they are irrelevant to whether those who are selected are the kinds of people they want clinicians to be. The question this criticism raises is: How do you select candidates who are caring and compassionate? Today, the answer is that we do not know, the same answer Flexner gave in 1910. If we do not know, it is not because the question has in theory and practice proved to be intractable. The fact is that the question has never been given the attention everybody seems to say is so necessary. Flexner at least said that the problem is an extraordinarily difficult one. One would have hoped that in the intervening decades the question would have stimulated a systematic research endeavor. But that never happened in medicine or in any of the other clinical fields. The problem is an extraordinarily difficult one, but since when does the level of difficulty excuse the absence of research? The absence of research, however, obscures a more simple and powerful factor: the unwillingness to experiment with admission criteria, an unwillingness that violates the morality of science. Once you change the criteria for admissions (or the allocation of weights to the different criteria) and once you test these criteria by the use of experimental and control groups—knowing ahead of time that you have embarked on uncharted seas—you have to be prepared to find out that you may have been wrong and that you have to go back to the conceptual drawing board.

Serious experimentation on admission criteria is no less than an effort to change some of the most important features of an organization, and it should occasion no surprise that the specter of such change engenders powerful resistances. Willingness to change has never been an obvious feature of individuals and organizations. As individuals and organizations, we like to do what we know how to do, and any suggestion of important change arouses fear of the unknown. So the suggestion that experimentation be done with new admission criteria is given short shrift, especially when these new criteria involve such "murky," hard-to-define concepts as caring and compassion. What gets lost sight of is that only when the problem is taken seriously will its theoretical and practical features gain clarity. The major goal of the research endeavor is to learn something that is important and replicable, accepting the maxim that the more you learn, the more you need to learn. In the current discussion, the significance of selection criteria has hardly been recognized as a scientific problem with enormous practical implications. What would require explanation would be if our clinical training centers in medicine, law, education, and psychology generally and sincerely embraced experimentation on admission criteria.

But there is another issue, no less thorny, that is important but has not surfaced. Let us assume that we have learned how better to select people who will be the kind of clinician we want them to be. How do we help them to capitalize on and enlarge their capacity to be caring and compassionate? I have already indicated that it is unrealistic to expect that courses and lectures are adequate means to achieve such a goal. It is not unrealistic to expect that the concept of mentors as models is more effective, but students encounter diverse models, many of whom are the opposite of what we want clinicians to be. What would be the characteristics of an appropriate model? How can such a model help the student other than by dependence on imitation not grounded in an explicit rational? In the next chapter, we will focus on a profession for which the central task is how to be caring and compassionate, a task that every one of the "clients" of that profession evaluates in the most explicit ways. Let us turn to the theater and actors.

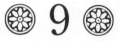

9

The Process
of Understanding:
The Relevance
of Stanislavski
for the Clinician

In the normal course of a day, we infrequently feel called upon to seek to understand another person's behavior. It would perhaps be more correct to say that we behave toward others as if we understood them. Most of our interactions bear the stamp of habit or ritual; that is, they are, for the most part, unthinking in that others take us and we take them without further probing, without questioning of ourselves or them. We and they may have covert agendas, and the focus is far more on completing agendas than on seeking understanding. It is not unusual for a person to go through an entire day without any interaction that is other than superficial: accepting surface appearances and verbalizations as necessary and sufficient for the purposes of the interactions. They are not interactions that "touch" us. Indeed, they are the symbolic polar opposites of "touching," because when we feel "touched," the interactions have been transformed into a transaction: they have changed something in us, and we feel the stirrings that will change something in others.

An example: Several years ago, I went to the local library, where I met an acquaintance whom I had not seen in some months. She was not what you would call a friend, but whenever we would meet, she and I would cheerily chat about this or that and then go our different ways. We liked each other, we would have liked to have been "real" friends, but time (always "time") and other excuses got in the way. So we met in the library and exchanged the usual greetings and questions: what books we had read recently, what books we were looking for, and so on. Habit and ritual dictated that we inquire about our spouses, and that is when she looked at me with surprise and asked: "You don't know that Gene died six weeks ago?" I was shocked, more than touched, because her husband was an unusually decent, sensitive human being whom I liked and respected. What stirred in me was less the fact of Gene's death and more the imagery of this woman alone in her lovely, large house faced with the task of reshaping her life. What if it were my wife in that situation? What should I, what could I say to this tearful woman that would make her feel I understood what she was up against? How could I be helpful? Our conversation changed dramatically. We were both touched and moved. What had begun as chitchat, the ritual (by no means unimportant) of courtesy and superficial interest, became for me a moment that obligated me to understand and help, to tear away the film of ritual and to seek a basis for help. The point is not whether I was helpful, or indulging a rescue fantasy, or possibly by my manner reopening a healing wound. The point is that I thought I understood, that I wanted to test that understanding for the purpose of being helpful. I could not be satisfied with uttering bromides.

Occasions that compel us to try to understand for the purpose of helping are not frequent. There are occasions that arouse us, mightily so, and cause us to try to understand ourselves and others, but they usually do not lead us to use that understanding to help another person. When they do, however, we become aware that, if arriving at understanding has problematic features, wedding that understanding appropriately to caring and compassionate actions is even more problematic, unless,

of course, one confuses intent with desired outcome. The process of understanding does not guarantee desired outcomes. It is
a necessary but not sufficient condition for action. Our understanding may be incomplete or faulty—it usually is—but that
does not necessarily mean that actions geared to helping will be
experienced by others as uncaring or uncompassionate. It is
often the case that others sense our desire to be caring and compassionate, and they appreciate our effort, but at the same time
they know that our actions fall far short of their mark. What
disturbs people, what makes the wall around them seem so im-
permeable, is their sense that helping actions are powered by
the language of social ritual and not by any real grappling with
the process of understanding. And that is the point: the process
of understanding is a grappling one that is manifested overtly in
ways that say "I am trying to understand because I want to be
helpful." It is those manifestations that are experienced as caring and compassionate, even though they may be more or less
ineffective. But when they are effective, the helper and helpee
are both changed.

    We like to see ourselves as caring and compassionate, but
people differ dramatically in their ability and willingness to
undertake the process of understanding in order to use those
feelings for appropriate actions. To *want* to understand implies
a commitment to action whose boundaries are necessarily unclear until one has reached the point where one feels that one
understands. If we resist that process, it is in part because we intuitively know that the commitment to action may involve pain
or inconvenience or self-sacrifice on our part; that is, we resist
the changes within us that understanding and a commitment to
action imply.

    If we are not born with the desire to understand or with
caring and compassionate feelings, we are far from comprehending why people come to differ so markedly in these respects. If the problem is a general one, it is of particular, practical significance for those responsible for selecting and training
clinicians. How does one sensitize clinicians of any stripe to the
nature and obligations of the caring role? I assume that no one
comes to the role, so to speak, fully formed and prepared. They

may come with all the right kinds of motivations, but that is clearly no guarantee that these motivations are integrated effectively with what is involved in understanding and action. What is required is a process of unlearning and learning, of giving up and acquiring, of seeing and using self in regard to others in altered ways.

The question I have raised has been most cogently, persuasively, and illuminatingly posed and discussed by Constantin Stanislavski (1936) in his book *An Actor Prepares*. It takes but a little reflection to recognize that the actor—any actor in any role, small or large—is faced with the task of becoming the role, of convincing us in the audience that he or she is the role. But we in the audience do not become aware that a role is being "played," that the actor has not become the role. This is particularly clear when we see a major actor about whose personal life we know a good deal and for whom we have a picture of the kind of person he or she is, of his or her life-style, or when, though we know very little about the actor's personal life, we have seen that actor in roles that "type" the person. We have a preformed picture of the person, and when we go to see that actor in a new production, we expect the role to convey that typing. If, however, the new role is quite different from the previous ones, we in the audience wonder whether that actor can convince us that he or she is the new role, that he or she has escaped from the confines of "typing," that we will not see the old in the new.

If this presents a problem for the audience, it presents an even greater problem for the actor. As an example, years ago we went to see the dramatic adaptation of Morris West's *The Devil's Advocate*, a novel about a priest with a terminal illness who is asked by the church to take on the role of the devil's advocate: to subject to the most critical scrutiny a proposal for the sanctification of an individual in a small town in Italy. The stance of the devil's advocate is that the presumed miracle or miracles being claimed for the person are explainable by means other than divine. It is a stance that requires both belief and disbelief. Now the actor we were to see in that role was Eduardo Cianelli, whom we had never seen on the stage but had seen in countless movies. And in every one of these movies, he played the Capone-like, surly, immoral gangster. If you knew that Eduardo Cianelli was going to be in a movie, you could describe his role ahead of time. If he was not the godfather, he was the loyal lieutenant. What was he doing in the role of West's devil's advocate, a role as far as one could imagine from any we had ever seen him in? And yet this turned out to be a peak experience in the theater for us. Within minutes after he came on stage, we forgot about the Eduardo Cianelli of the movies. Indeed, we forgot about Eduardo Cianelli. He *was* the role. There was no cleavage between the person and the role.

How does an actor become the role? What is the process whereby an actor strives to understand another person, that is, the role? Why do actors, especially the neophytes, so vastly underestimate or bypass that process of understanding? What are the predictable obstacles the actor has to overcome if the nature and ramifications of the role are to be comprehended, especially if the role is one that is foreign to the life experiences of the actor, as is usually the case, as was the case with Cianelli? These are the questions, among others, that Stanislavski takes up. Forget that the book is about actors. Wherever the word *actor* appears, you could substitute the word *clinician* without changing Stanislavski's rationale or the book as a major psychological treatise illuminating the dynamics of caring and compassionate action.[1] How do you understand and become another person when that person is so different from you, and, despite the difference, how do you imaginatively use personal events and memories to bridge that difference? Granted that

---

[1] I am not, of course, suggesting that actors are clinicians, that actors have the same relationships to their roles that clinicians have to their clients. But I am asserting that clinicians and actors have the task of understanding someone else on his or her own terms and that such understanding cannot be achieved without being caring and compassionate. Clearly, the desire to be caring and compassionate is, by itself, no guarantee that understanding appropriate to the desired outcome will be achieved. What is so instructive about Stanislavski is the way he demonstrates how the process of understanding interconnects caring and compassion, personal experience, "objective" knowledge, and what I would call the freedom to imagine.

your background and outlook are not those of Hamlet, how do you imaginatively use personal events, memories, and lived experience as a basis for understanding what Hamlet is and feels? One cannot read Stanislavski without the questions multiplying, because what he has to say is in principle so apposite to the role of the clinician.

An Actor Prepares is extraordinarily concrete in that each point Stanislavski makes is illustrated with examples. The reader is never left in doubt about what Stanislavski means. Furthermore, Stanislavski uses a series of examples in order to convey the developmental nature of the process of understanding a role. Understanding does not come full blown but rather is a result of grappling with three major obstacles: underestimating the scope and complexity of the process, failure to use one's own life experiences creatively, and resistance to the idea that the process is a never-ending one. What keeps the actor engaged in what is a demanding cognitive and affective process and quest? The answer is that the actor cares for the other person (the role) and seeks compassionately to identify with and to become the other person. That person may be hateful, unlovable, destructive, and evil, but the actor's task is to understand that person to the degree that the actor willingly and compassionately makes that person's phenomenology convincing to an audience. The actor cannot indulge his or her prejudices or values; that is, the actor cannot dislike the person. Strange to say, the actor must care for and be compassionate toward that person if the actor is to become that person. In "real life," the actor may recoil from anyone with the characteristics of an Iago, but when he seeks to play that role, he cares for Iago. You cannot "become" somebody for whom you have no feelings of caring and compassion. When one actor says that he can play Iago better than another actor, he is saying that he understands Iago better, that he is more sensitive to nuances in Iago's character and outlook, that he cares more for Iago: he has probed more deeply for the roots of Iago's thinking and behavior so that he can feel he is Iago. When an actor says he loves a certain role, there is a part of that actor that means it literally, however revolting that role is to the audience.

At the time I was writing this chapter, an article by
Samuel G. Freedman (1984) appeared in the drama section of
the *New York Times*. The following are excerpts from the
article:

When actors move audiences in "After the
Fall," the achievement has not come cheaply. The
play is one of the most daring and troublesome in
the Arthur Miller canon, a tale of a lawyer's failures at love, of his pain and self-pity, told through
a mosaic of scenes. It is compelling to some, con-
founding to others.

But there has been little dissent about the
starring performances of Frank Langella and Diane
Wiest in the revival of "After the Fall" now at
Playhouse 91. In a drama that makes people uncomfortable—and that is its strength as well as its
weakness—they have won the applause of both critics and audiences.

That success may have come in part because
Mr. Langella, Miss Wiest and the director John Tillinger confronted, even embraced, the disquieting
nature of the play. Mr. Langella's Quentin and Miss
Wiest's Maggie emerge less as heroes or victims than
as complex beings—wounded and wounding, vulnerable and self-absorbed.

"It could be the single worst trap for an actor to want to be liked," Mr. Langella said. "It's a
stultifying insecurity. It's in me, it's in all of us,
and we must fight it. To want to be liked is to ultimately compromise. You begin to live for other
people. It shouldn't rule your life and it shouldn't
rule the roles you play. I have failed as Quentin
whenever I overplayed the sympathetic side. Whenever I tried to entertain, I lost the audience." . . .

"This play doesn't need any defending," he
said. "People complain about Quentin comparing
his pain to the pain of the Jews in the Holocaust.

But isn't the real honesty that we *are* most concerned about our own pain? Our conceit is that we
feel first about the pain of the world."

While Mr. Langella knew for years he would
play Quentin, Miss Wiest had not even read the
play until the audition. . . . She was the 35th woman to try for the part, but she won it on one reading.

A peculiar kind of chemistry quickly
emerged. On the second or third day of rehearsals,
Mr. Langella started talking about the "plight" of
Quentin. The actresses who play Quentin's wives
and lovers, among them Miss Wiest, shouted him
down. Mr. Langella, worried, asked Mr. Tillinger,
"What are we going to do?" The director replied,
"They're playing their parts."

Later in the rehearsals, Miss Wiest found it
increasingly difficult to play the scenes in which
Maggie attempts suicide and Quentin tries to stran-
gle her. "We all felt this incredible reluctance to go
into the play," she recalled. "I was scared of the
pain." One afternoon, she simply wept through the
entire suicide scene. . . .

"I think Maggie and Quentin have the arche-
typal magnetism between a guilty intellectual and a
passionate, self-indulgent, self-destructive person,"
Miss Wiest said. "That magnetism could have a
healthy side, but for Maggie and Quentin the guilt
and the self-destruction feed on each other. Yet
right to the end, the love is there, because of the
need each has for the other." . . .

In playing Quentin, Mr. Langella turned to
the playwright—who shared memories and letters
with him—and into himself. "The more I peeled
away the layers, the more I saw myself," he said.
"With certain scripts you read, bells go off. I'm
44 now, maybe five, six years behind Quentin. And
this play's about how a man that age begins to in-

vestigate his past and tries to avoid his past mis-
takes. As you grow older and have children, as you
become a father as well as a son, you begin to ask
yourself different questions.

"Quentin is a man on a quest. I'm sure, in
fact, that's why Arthur named him Quentin. And
playing him is difficult in the same sense the play is
difficult to take; you're asking an awful lot of
yourself and the people around you to face this
murderous instinct, this need to survive everything.
It's the same reason this play has as many de-
tractors as supporters."

One of the hallmarks of great professionals is that they
make their performances seem easy, so easy at times that we
can imagine ourselves imitating them. We think we can imitate
them, unaware that what we have seen is a result of a struggle to
understand another person in his or her complexity; that is, the
kind of background from which that person emerged, the way
of looking at self and others, the mixture of motivations their
actions reflect and suggest. To imitate actions is one thing; to
make them believable is quite another thing, and that is the
point Freedman is making and the point that Stanislavski so
brilliantly illuminates. And, I must repeat, believability comes
from a struggle in which, caringly and compassionately, one
seeks understanding of another person. When Wiest says that
one afternoon she simply wept through the entire suicide scene,
she is not seeking our sympathy or revealing her personal vul-
nerabilities or being bathetic. She is describing a necessary struggle. And when Langella says "I have failed as Quentin whenever
I have overplayed the sympathetic side. Whenever I tried to entertain, I lost the audience," he is telling us, as Stanislavski emphasizes, that the struggle is a never-ending one. We in the audience are spared that struggle, unless the performance is so bad
that we undertake to try to understand what is taking place,
and why, on the stage. Then we have an inkling, the barest inkling, of what Stanislavski means by "the actor prepares."

It could be argued that in comparing actors and clinicians

I am confusing the *appearance* of compassion (*seeming* to be interested and compassionate) on the part of actors with the actual *presence* of compassion on the part of clinicians. My reading of Stanislavski, as well as of the introspections of actors, is that when acting a part the actor becomes the role, although there are always fleeting moments when they are aware of themselves. Those fleeting moments, however, do not make the process psychologically fraudulent. If anything, those moments reflect the necessary boundaries, for actors and clinicians, that control against the dangers of excesses that can come from fusion of self with other. Yes, the clinician, like the actor, runs the risk of overinvolvement but surely to reduce that risk by underinvolvement is to substitute one excess for another.

But now we come to what I consider Stanislavski's greattest insight. It is one of those insights that when articulated seems a glimpse of the obvious, but how frequently do we take the obvious seriously? The actor prepares for a particular role, and it is understandable if he or she rivets on that single role (just as the clinician rivets on the palpable person before him or her). But that role is integrally related to all other roles in the play. Can you understand a role as if it were independent of the other roles? Can you understand Iago independent of Othello or Desdemona? Is the phenomenology of one comprehensible apart from that of the others? Can the actor avoid dealing with the interdependence of roles? Concretely and ingeniously, Stanislavski illustrates why the actor should not, must not, see his or her role apart from the others. Can you understand a member of a family without seeing that person in the truly seamless psychological web of all members of the family? Long before the theoretical and practical rationale of family therapy was developed, Stanislavski had formulated the rationale and its educational-training implications. And, as was the case with family therapy, what was at stake for Stanislavski was how to improve outcomes, how this enlarged conception of the obligations of the actor would make for a more powerfully moving performance. What Stanislavski sought to inculcate in his students was an attitude of caring toward all roles in the play.

It has not been my intention to examine or review Stanislavski's theory and "method." My intention was twofold. First, I wanted to indicate that in a field seemingly far removed from and, on the surface, completely unrelated to the clinical endeavor, Stanislavski had made understanding, caring, and compassion central issues. And in doing so, he illuminated not only their centrality but the obstacles with which mentors and students had to struggle if the process of understanding, caring, and compassion was appropriately to inform action. How to understand another person in the context of that person's interpersonal drama—not as a single, isolated organism, not as one who is unaffected by or in turn has no effects on others in his or her family drama—that is what Stanislavski illuminated, and the theater has never been the same since.[2] The second of my intentions was to indicate that Stanislavski did not stay on the level of theory but developed an educational rationale that sought to help the actor become more aware of how self is both asset and liability, of how self in the normal course of living is unmined as a source of understanding others, of how one's own history is both protagonist and antagonist, so to speak, in comprehending others with histories markedly different from one's own. An actor (like the clinician) cannot afford to dislike a role he or she willingly assumes; the actor has to strive to "touch" the role so that others are "touched"; the actor seeks understanding for the purpose of action appropriate to that understanding; the actor has to learn the difference between becom-

[2]To want to understand requires, among other things, integrating two sources of knowledge. The first source is what you think you know about the person in the here and now, what you decide is factual or has a high probability of being factual. The second source is formal knowledge (always intertwined with personal experience, judgment, and interpretation) that, so to speak, says: "When you observe certain facts in the here and now, you are dealing with this and not that condition and, therefore, this is the way you should or should not proceed." The greater the clinician's experience and formal knowledge, the more respect the clinician has for the importance of deciding what is factual in the here and now. At least that is what we assume happens with experience. But to what extent does that "practice makes perfect" assumption hold? If I ask that question in regard to understanding, caring, and compassion, it is to suggest again that we can no longer be satisfied with answers that confuse assumption with demonstration, passionate beliefs with empirically based conclusions.

ing a symptom and becoming the person who has the symptom
(for example, Othello's jealousy).

I did not bring Stanislavski into this discussion in any
way to suggest that his educational methods should be applied
to the training of clinicians. That his methods have (or will be
found to have) potential, practical relevance to such training I
have no doubt whatsoever. How and at what point in clinical
training Stanislavski's point of view can be introduced and
adapted I cannot say. Furthest from my mind is the hope that
those who may see the relevance of Stanislavski for clinical
training will push for curriculum reform. Stanislavski is no
panacea, just as psychoanalysis, behavior modification, and drug
therapies have been no panaceas. What Stanislavski gives us is an
elaborated point of view from which he developed a method of
instruction. For the clinical professions it is, at this time, his
point of view that needs to be understood, its relevance for clinicians thought through, possible methodologies outlined, and
systematic investigation and evaluation of whatever actions are
taken carried out. We have no need of nostrums. What we need
is clarity of view, a willingness to experiment, and an appreciation for the fact that, as with any other problem scientifically
approached, we can expect that the more we learn, the more we
will need to learn. Let us not get into curriculum reform without that sense of security that comes from no-holds-barred in-
vestigations that take the sting out of the criticism that a pas-
sionately held point of view is no substitute for an empirical
test. And therein lies a major problem: that criticism is valid for
the beliefs that *currently* undergird clinical training in the diverse professions I have discussed. As I emphasized earlier, not
only are these beliefs assumed to be valid, natural, and proper
but they are the justifications for opposing alternative points of
view. The relevance of Stanislavski for clinicians? One does not
have to be very imaginative to predict that most of those who
so tenaciously cling to the beliefs that inform current clinical
training curricula will view that question either with staring disbelief or with that polite tolerance that the frivolous fantasies
of serious but misguided idealists should be accorded. It is both
understandable and wise to resist succumbing to every new idea

one is pressured to assimilate and implement. What is unwise is to fail to distinguish between the problem and the new ideas it addresses and the method offered for solution. So, for example, when Freud developed his concept of the death instinct, many people derided his effort at the same time that they glossed over the fact that he was addressing a momentous problem: how to explain the origins and vicissitudes of aggressive behavior.

If I appear gun-shy about implementing Stanislavski's point of view, and about the modal way in which curriculum reform is carried out, it is an accurate perception. Let me give the most recent example that gives force to my hesitations. In the drama section of the *New York Times* for April 15, 1985, there was an article entitled "O'Neill Performed for Mayo Doctors." Several actors (Jason Robards, Sam Robards, Teresa Wright, Margaret Hunt) performed and read scenes from Eugene O'Neill's *Long Day's Journey into Night*. The scenes dealt with the narcotic addiction of Mary Tyrone, the wife, and the reactions of her family. The audience was 1600 staff physicians, residents, and personnel of the Mayo Clinic and Foundation. The occasion was the fourth in an "Insight" series undertaken in 1981 to study human behavior through the medium of the theater. The director of the series explained: "We call the program 'Insight' because it is not to give answers but to give insight into the common human problems that are a great part of every physician's practice, but a small part of his or her education. Physicians don't need any more facts, and the time they can spend on human problems, their own and others, is very limited. The theater can move into that gap." One Mayo professor is quoted as saying: "We are a group of physicians who are highly subspecialized. But even for general practitioners, there is almost no formal training in subjects like alcoholism, drug addiction, aging, and suicide. Many physicians feel ill-prepared and incompetent in these areas." Another professor said: "This allows physicians to see these problems from a different aspect; we tend to see them in a more clinical way." Finally, another professor states: "One danger we have is becoming accustomed to our own methodology and not being terribly flexible in seeing things from the view of other people."

The rationale for the series requires comment. For one thing, it explicitly recognizes that physicians are deficient in their understanding of people with a chemical dependency, or who are old, or who seek to end their lives. It also recognizes that neither in their medical education nor in their practice do they have the time to gain an understanding of such "common problems." There is a third feature that I will address after discussing this question: what are the objectives of the series? I shall assume that, although the audience enjoyed the presentation, enjoyment was not a major goal. Clearly, the audience is to gain a broadened and deepened understanding of people presumably quite different from themselves, an understanding leading to and becoming intertwined with feelings of caring and compassion. Stated in this way, it is an objective to be attained not only by this audience but by any audience that sees this stirring play; that was O'Neill's objective. But this series is not meant to be simply a night in the theater watching superb actors illuminate the phenomenology of ill people. This play was presented to an audience of physicians presumably for the purpose of deepening their understanding in order to influence their subsequent actions with their patients. This, of course, raises two questions. What understanding did these medical personnel attain? How will such an understanding inform their actions? We do not and cannot know the answers to these questions. After all, the series is intended "to fill a gap," to make a difference in the way these physicians understand and act. Can one assume that they will get the "proper" understanding, that it will "appropriately" inform their behavior? I am not suggesting that this series should have been embedded in a research project. I use the series as an example of how an educational issue can be recognized and then dealt with in a superficial manner that obscures rather than illuminates the ramifications of the issue, and, significantly, in a way that provides no empirical basis for learning more about an issue that all concerned admit is a crucial one. The Mayo Clinic did not achieve its reputation by researching important problems in this way, by starting with belief and hope and ending with belief and hope. But, one might ask, is not the series better than nothing? My answer is in the negative because it gives the appearance of appropriateness at the expense of trivializing, if not burying, the problem. And that brings me to the third aspect of the rationale for the series: the assumption that, despite the deficits in medical education with regard to people who are drug dependent, aged, or suicidal, physicians have the appropriate understanding, caring, and compassionate approach toward the patients they encounter in their specialties. The series does not and cannot challenge this assumption. But this series does have one clear virtue: it approaches, albeit incompletely and indirectly, recognition of a significant issue.

The problem today in regard to clinical training is not one of method or curriculum but rather of facing squarely what we mean when we say that clinicians should be more caring and compassionate than they are. And that is where Stanislavski comes in, where he is directly relevant, where he has presented us with the dilemmas and opportunities, where what he says about understanding, caring, and compassion illuminates the problem and we literally see it in a new light. We can no longer be satisfied with remedies in the form of courses and lectures that derive from the grossest oversimplifications of the nature of caring and compassion. Clinicians are not actors, but both have a good deal in common. Stanislavski writes about actors, but this does not validate the claim that what he has to say has limited generality. It is true that, in illuminating the issues, he has made the task of the actor more demanding and complex, but since when is simplicity an inherent virtue? It is also true that, if we were to take Stanislavski even half seriously, it would require a very discernible change in how we prepare clinicians. When a problem is redefined, it understandably meets resistance in those whose actions are informed by traditional patterns of thought. The redefiners, and Stanislavski is one, should not expect that those whose thinking they seek to influence will roll out the welcome mat. Stanislavski's theory and practice met, and continue to meet, resistance in many quarters in the theater, although over the years his rationale seems to have become part of the conventional wisdom.

It would be understandable to me if clinicians, or the

teachers of clinicians, who read Stanislavski would be critical or would at least have great difficulty imagining how his seminal ideas could be applied in clinical training programs that are now so full of requirements that altering them in meaningful ways should be undertaken only by those with untapped reservoirs of masochistic needs. What would be inexcusable to me would be if Stanislavski—more specifically, the kinds of issues he raised—remained foreign, indeed unknown, to those well-meaning educators concerned with a perceived determination in the caring and compassionate actions of clinicians. You cannot read Stanislavski, if you are a teacher of clinicians, and then blithely resume customary ways of thinking. Actors are not clinicians, just as tomatoes are not apples, yet the elements in these two pairs share underlying similarities, if not identities. So we have a basis for saying that apples and tomatoes are both fruit, just as we are justified in saying that clinicians and actors both engage in a process involving caring, compassion, and the quest for understanding.

This theme of surface differences and underlying commonalities is identical to one I discussed in earlier chapters where I endeavored to show that (some) lawyers and teachers have kinship with physicians in general and psychiatrists in particular and with clinical psychologists. It is perhaps not happenstance that, in the modern world (which began a long time ago), the forces that have weakened the bonds that keep people together—that make them feel socially connected—are the forces that further weaken the always fragile connections among different fields of knowledge and inquiry. Labels are not the "cause" of this weakening, but, once labels take hold, they become an almost insuperable obstacle to the perception of commonalities. So, when we hear much these days about the lack of caring and compassion among physicians, there is little to warn us that physicians are but one of the groups that comprise the clinical endeavor. And when, in the context of discussing the clinical endeavor, I plead that Stanislavski's point of view be given a serious hearing, I hope that the fact that he talks about acting will not be used as justification for ignoring him.

A final comment about the relevance of Stanislavski. In

earlier chapters, I emphasized how in practice the stance of the clinician is toward the single individual and that failure to understand how the problems that person presents affect others around him or her, and how they in turn transactionally affect the person, robs the clinician of the opportunity to prevent problems. The hallmark of the clinical endeavor is that the clinician is confronted with someone in some kind of distress. The source of the distress may be known or unknown, but there is a problem, and the clinician endeavors to relieve the distress. But the problems of people almost always (one should assume always) have direct significance for others with whom the person is related, and it is in relation to those significances that the opportunity for preventive action arises. As long as the clinician ignores those significances—as long as the clinician focuses narrowly on *the* problem in *the* single individual—the opportunity for preventive actions cannot be recognized and seized. Can an actor understand a role independent of the other roles? In posing and discussing that question, Stanislavski gives us a rationale relevant to how clinicians should look at people and their problems. The clinical and preventive endeavors are not antitheses. The stance of one is not inimical to the other. The fact is that in practice, and the ways clinicians are prepared for practice, the preventive stance is conspicuous by its absence.

The clinical endeavor has come under public scrutiny as never before. I suppose that it has long been the case that clinicians and those they seek to help have been in a love-hate relationship. To seek help is to arouse strong and conflicting feelings, not the least of which are fear and the need to be understood and cared about and for. In seeking help, we need and expect a lot from another human being, often to such an extent as to guarantee disappointment. Although this is well understood by many clinicians, it engenders discomfort in them, because they are sensitive to their limitations in knowledge and skill. There are, of course, clinicians who bask in the attributes of the role of a divinity that their clients so frequently project onto them. They are, in my experience, a minority of clinicians. Far more numerous are clinicians who know that, for one reason or another, they are unadept in the matter of understanding their clients and seeing and dealing with the social-familial ramifications of their problems. That feeling of the lack of adeptness is something of which the beginning clinician is quite aware. The expectation, on our or their parts, is, of course, that with experience their adeptness will increase. In the narrow technical sense, that may well happen, but in regard to the issues I have raised in this book, cumulative experience is far from a corrective. Quite the contrary; unprepared as they are by their training in these matters, their sensitivities—what Flexner called their "requisite insight and sympathy"—tend to become more blunted, rationalized away on the basis of the pressures of time and economics and the boundaries of specialization in knowledge and role. And that situation has to be understood in light of the fact that the criteria by which people are selected into clinical professions are literally irrelevant to the goal of selecting people who are or have the potential to become caring and compassionate clinicians. In practice, the processes of selection and self-selection rely on Lady Luck to achieve the desired objectives, but it has long been apparent, as current concerns and reports testify, that Lady Luck has not been on our side.

Yes, the problem is, as Flexner said, an admittedly difficult one, but that does not excuse, if only on scientific grounds, the paucity of research on the issues surrounding selection and self-selection. When Flexner said the problem was difficult, he could just as well have said in 1910 that going to the moon was a difficult, if not impossible, problem to tackle, let alone to solve even partially. But we got to the moon, and for two reasons. First, within the scientific community, there were some people who were gripped by the problem and its potential significances, scientific and otherwise. They stayed with the problem. Second, it became in the national interest to pursue space exploration; that is, it became more than a scientific problem. The problem of selection and self-selection for the clinical endeavor has been neglected by the clinical professions and cannot be said to occupy an important place in the national interest. In a vague, inchoate way, people feel and know that the clinical endeavor has become problematic, that those who are in helping

roles are both cause and victim, that something is wrong somewhere, and that, far from getting better, it seems to be getting
worse, that as the objects of help they are indeed "objects" and
not persons.

It is clear from what I have said in these pages that I believe that the remedies currently being offered, however well intentioned, obscure rather than clarify the issues. Indeed, the
fact that the issues are currently being raised only in relation to
medical clinicians is a reflection of how narrowly the clinical
endeavor is defined. It is a narrowness of view that our society
can no longer afford if we are to give more than lip service to
the superiority of prevention over repair. Abraham Flexner pre-
sided over the wedding between science and medicine. We must
await the societal conditions from which will emerge another
Abraham Flexner who will preside over the wedding between
prevention and the clinical endeavor. The first wedding reflected and gave rise to individual and institutional turmoil and
transformations. Individuals and institutions do not greet
change warmly, to understate matters extremely. The second
wedding is and will be no exception.

References

American Psychiatric Association. *Psychiatry and Medical Education. Report of the Conference on Psychiatric Education.* Washington, D.C.: American Psychiatric Association, 1952.

American Psychiatric Association. *The Psychiatrist: His Training and Development. Report of the Conference on Psychiatric Education.* Washington, D.C.: American Psychiatric Association, 1953.

Association of American Medical Colleges. *Physicians for the Twenty-First Century: Report of the Panel on the General Education of the Physician and College Preparation for Medicine.* Washington, D.C.: Association of American Medical Colleges, 1984.

Baird, M. "The Physician as Therapist." *Family Networker,* 1985, *9* (1), 31.

Beers, C. W. *A Mind That Found Itself.* New York: Doubleday, Doran, 1928.

Blatt, B. *Exodus from Pandemonium.* Boston: Allyn & Bacon, 1970.

Block, C. B. "Diagnostic and Treatment Issues for Black Patients." *Clinical Psychologist,* 1984, *37* (2), 51-54.

Bok, D. "Needed: A New Way to Train Doctors." *Harvard Magazine,* May-June 1984, pp. 32-43.

Boyd-Franklin, N. "Issues in Family Therapy with Black Families." *Clinical Psychologist,* 1984, *37* (2), 54-59.

Deutsch, A. *The Shame of the States.* New York: Harcourt Brace Jovanovich, 1948.

Deutsch, A. *The Mentally Ill in America.* New York: Columbia University Press, 1949.

Doane, J., and Cowen, E. "Interpersonal Help-Giving of Family Practice Lawyers." *American Journal of Community Psychology,* 1981, *9* (5), 547-558.

Dollard, J. *Criteria for the Life History.* New Haven: Yale University Press, 1935.

Dym, B., and Berman, S. "Family Systems Medicine: Family Therapy's Next Frontier?" *Family Networker,* 1985, *9* (1), 20.

Eisenberg, L. "The Search for Care." *Daedalus,* 1977, *106* (1), 235-246.

Engel, G. I. "The Need for a New Medical Model." *Science,* 1977, *196,* 129-136.

Featherstone, H. *A Difference in the Family: Life with a Disabled Child.* New York: Basic Books, 1980.

Federman, D. D. "Can Compassion Survive?" *Stanford, M.D.,* 1975, *14* (3), 14-16.

Flexner, A. *I Remember: The Autobiography of Abraham Flexner.* New York: Simon & Schuster, 1940.

Flexner, A. *Medical Education in the United States and Canada: A Report to the Carnegie Foundation for the Advancement of Teaching.* Washington, D.C.: Carnegie Foundation for the Advancement of Teaching, 1960. (Originally published 1910.)

Freedman, S. G. "Wiest and Langella Play Complex Roles in 'Fall.' " *New York Times,* Nov. 5, 1984.

Gladwin, T. *Slaves of the White Myth: The Psychology of Neocolonialism.* Atlantic Highlands, N.J.: Humanities Press, 1980.

Glenn, M. "The Therapist in Medical Practice." *Family Networker,* 1985, *9* (1), 30.

Goldhammer, R. *Clinical Supervision.* New York: Holt, Rinehart and Winston, 1969.

Gordon, S., and Steele, R. E. "Consultation and the Mental Health of Minority Communities: An Examination of the Literature from 1973 Through 1983." *Newsletter of the Divi-*

sion of Community Psychology (American Psychological Association), 1984, *17* (2), 4–5.

Grob, G. W. *Mental Illness and American Society, 1875–1940.* Princeton, N.J.: Princeton University Press, 1983.

Harris, C. *One Man's Medicine.* New York: Harper & Row, 1975.

Hechinger, F. "Medical Text Revives Lost Skill: Compassion." *New York Times,* July 31, 1984.

Heifetz, L. J. "From Consumer to Middleman: Emerging Roles for Parents in the Network of Services for Retarded Children." In R. R. Abidian (ed.), *Parent Education and Intervention Handbook.* Springfield, Ill.: Thomas, 1980.

Hochschild, A. R. *The Managed Heart: Commercialization of Human Feelings.* Berkeley: University of California Press, 1983.

Huang, L. N., and Heifetz, L. J. "Elements of Professional Helpfulness." Paper presented at the Sixth International Congress of the International Association for the Scientific Study of Mental Deficiency, Toronto, 1982.

"Interpersonal Relations in Health Care." *Journal of Social Issues,* 1975 (entire issue no. 1).

Jones, E. E. "Some Reflections on the Black Patient and Psychotherapy." *Clinical Psychologist,* 1984, *37* (2), 62–65.

Jones, J. M., and Block, C. B. "Black Cultural Perspectives." *Clinical Psychologist,* 1984, *37* (2), 58–62.

Katz, J. *The Silent World of Doctor and Patient.* New York: Free Press, 1984.

Kennedy, D. *Legal Education and the Reproduction of Hierarchy.* Cambridge, Mass.: Afar, 1983.

Lenrow, P. B., and Burch, R. M. "Mutual and Professional Services: Opposing or Complementary?" In B. Gottlieb (ed.), *Networks and Social Support.* New York: Sage, 1981.

Levine, M. *The History and Politics of Community Mental Health.* New York: Oxford University Press, 1981.

"MacNeil-Lehrer News Hour. Physician, Heal Thyself." Sept. 6, 1984, transcript no. 2334, pp. 10–13.

Maeroff, G. "Broader Education for Medical Students Proposed." *New York Times,* Sept. 20, 1984.

Margolick, D. "The Trouble with America's Law Schools." *New York Times Magazine,* May 22, 1983, pp. 20-25.

Marsh, A. "Attitudes Toward the Refusal of Life-Enhancing Help or Treatment." Doctoral dissertation, Department of Psychology, Yale University, 1985.

Martinez, F. H. "A Manager's View of Hispanic Mental Health Care in the Community." *Newsletter of the Division of Community Psychology* (American Psychological Association), 1984, *17* (2), 6-7.

Mayhew, K. C., and Edwards, A. C. *The Dewey School.* New York: Atherton Press, 1966.

Merton, R. K., Reader, G., and Kendall, P. L. (eds.) *The Student-Physician.* Cambridge, Mass.: Harvard University Press, 1957.

Nelson, R. "Can Doctors Learn Warmth?" *New York Times,* Sept. 13, 1983, Science Section, p. 1.

Pellegrino, E. D. "Educating the Humanist Physician." *Journal of the American Medical Association,* 1974, *222,* 1288-1294.

Raimy, V. (ed.). *Training in Clinical Psychology.* Englewood Cliffs, N.J.: Prentice-Hall, 1950.

Reiser, D. E., and Rosen, D. H. *Medicine as a Human Experience.* Baltimore: University Park Press, 1984.

Reppucci, N. D., Weithorn, L. A., Mulvey, E. P., and Monahan, J. (eds.). *Children, Mental Health, and the Law.* Vol. 4. Beverly Hills, Calif.: Sage Publications, 1984.

Richardson, H. B. *Patients Have Families.* New York: Commonwealth Fund, 1945.

Riessman, F. "Self-helpers." *Nation,* June 2, 1984.

Roemer, M. I. "Prospects of Ambulatory Health Care and Their Meaning for Allied Health Personnel." *New York University Education Quarterly,* Spring/Summer 1983, pp. 17-22.

Sarason, S. B. *Psychological Problems in Mental Deficiency.* New York: Harper & Row, 1949.

Sarason, S. B. *The Psychological Sense of Community: Prospects for a Community Psychology.* San Francisco: Jossey-Bass, 1974.

Sarason, S. B. *Work, Aging, and Social Change: Professionals and the One-Life-One-Career Imperative.* New York: Free Press, 1977.

Sarason, S. B. "An Asocial Psychology and a Misdirected Clinical Psychology." *American Psychologist,* 1981, *36* (8), 827-836.

Sarason, S. B. *The Culture of the School and the Problem of Change.* Boston: Allyn & Bacon, 1982.

Sarason, S. B. *Schooling in America.* New York: Free Press, 1983.

Sarason, S. B. *The Psychology of Mental Retardation.* Austin, Tex.: Pro-Ed, 1985.

Sarason, S. B., Davidson, K., and Blatt, B. *The Preparation of Teachers: An Unstudied Problem in Education.* New York: Wiley, 1960.

Sarason, S. B., and Doris, J. *Educational Handicap, Public Policy, and Social History.* New York: Free Press, 1979.

Sarason, S. B., and Klaber, M. "The School as a Social Situation." *Annual Review of Psychology,* 1985, *36,* 115-140.

Sarason, S. B., Sarason, E. K., and Cowden, P. "Aging and the Nature of Work." *American Psychologist,* 1975, *30* (5), 584-592.

Shore, M. F. "Marking Time in the Land of Plenty: Reflections on Mental Health in the United States." *American Journal of Orthopsychiatry,* 1981, *51* (3), 391-402.

Silver, G. A. *A Spy in the House of Medicine.* Germantown, Md.: Aspen Systems, 1976.

Stanislavski, C. *An Actor Prepares.* New York: Theater Arts Books, 1936.

Starr, P. *The Discarded Army: Veterans After Vietnam.* New York: Charterhouse, 1974.

Starr, P. *The Social Transformation of American Medicine.* New York: Basic Books, 1982.

Stevens, R., and Stevens, R. *Welfare Medicine in America: A Case Study of Medicaid.* New York: Free Press, 1974.

Stone, E. S. "The Adoption of Handicapped Children." Doctoral dissertation, Department of Psychology, Yale University, 1982.

Thomas, L. *The Youngest Science.* New York: Viking Press, 1983.

Turnbull, A. P., and Turnbull, H. R. (eds.). *Parents Speak Out.* Columbus, Ohio: Merrill, 1979.

Veblen, T. *The Higher Learning in America: A Memorandum on the Conduct of Universities by Business Men.* New York: Sagamore Books, 1957. (Originally published 1918.)

Wahl, S. *The Medical Industrial Complex.* New York: Harmony Books, 1984.

Wolfensberger, W., and Kurtz, R. A. (eds.). *Management of the Family of the Mentally Retarded.* Chicago: Follett Educational Corporation, 1969.

Zigler, E., and Valentine, J. *Project Head Start: Success or Failure?* New York: Free Press, 1979.

Index